AF379040

Series in BioEngineering

Series Editor

Magdalena Stoeva, Medical Imaging Department, Medical University Plovdiv, Plovdiv, Bulgaria

The Series in Bioengineering serves as an information source for a professional audience in science and technology as well as for advanced students. It covers all applications of the physical sciences and technology to medicine and the life sciences. Its scope ranges from bioengineering, biomedical and clinical engineering to biophysics, biomechanics, biomaterials, and bioinformatics.

Indexed by WTI Frankfurt eG, zbMATH.

Almir Badnjević • Lemana Spahić

Biosensors

Principles, Technologies, and Emerging Innovations

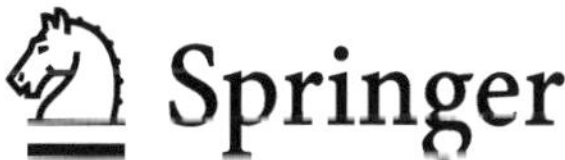 Springer

Almir Badnjević
Registers and Data Exchange of B & H
Agency for Identification Documents
Banja Luka, Bosnia and Herzegovina

Lemana Spahić ⓘD
Research Institute Verlab
Sarajevo, Bosnia and Herzegovina

ISSN 2196-8861   ISSN 2196-887X (electronic)
Series in BioEngineering
ISBN 978-3-032-15756-0   ISBN 978-3-032-15757-7 (eBook)
https://doi.org/10.1007/978-3-032-15757-7

This Springer imprint is published by the registered company Springer Nature Switzerland AG
The registered company address is: Gewerbestrasse 11, 6330 Cham, Switzerland

If disposing of this product, please recycle the paper.

Foreword

This textbook provides a structured introduction to biosensors, covering their fundamental principles, diverse applications, and the latest advancements in biosensing technologies. It is designed for students, researchers, and professionals in biomedical engineering, analytical chemistry, and sensor technology.

This book begins with an introduction to biosensors, defining their classification, historical evolution, and key components, such as biorecognition elements, transduction mechanisms, and signal processing techniques. Applications in healthcare, environmental monitoring, and industrial settings are also explored.

A detailed section on biosensor fundamentals covers biorecognition strategies using enzymes, antibodies, nucleic acids, and molecular imprinting. Signal transduction mechanisms, including electrochemical, optical, and acoustic techniques, are discussed alongside key performance parameters, such as selectivity, sensitivity, and response time. The challenges and limitations of biosensors in real-world applications are also examined.

This book introduces measurement uncertainty in biosensors, addressing sources of variability, calibration methods, and statistical error analysis. The ISO Guide to the Expression of Uncertainty in Measurement (ISO GUM) is discussed, providing methodologies for uncertainty quantification and budgeting with practical case studies.

A comprehensive exploration of different biosensor types follows, including electrochemical biosensors for glucose monitoring and drug analysis, optical biosensors using fluorescence and surface plasmon resonance (SPR) for medical diagnostics and food safety, and impedance biosensors for cellular analysis and cancer detection. Additional sections cover acoustic and piezoelectric biosensors, field-effect transistor (FET)-based biosensors, and cutting-edge nanotechnology-enhanced immunosensors.

This book also examines biomedical applications of biosensors, such as disease diagnostics, personalized medicine, wearable biosensors, drug discovery, and lab-on-a-chip integration. A concluding section on future trends and challenges discusses advancements in nanomaterials, artificial intelligence-driven biosensor data analysis, regulatory considerations, and the integration of smart biosensors with the Internet of Things (IoT).

Blending theoretical foundations with real-world applications, this textbook serves as a comprehensive guide for understanding biosensors and their transformative impact across scientific and healthcare domains.

Siena, Italy   Ernesto Iadanza

Preface

This textbook provides a comprehensive introduction to biosensors, integrating foundational principles, measurement methodologies, and modern technological advancements with a particular focus on biomedical and analytical applications. It is intended for students, researchers, and professionals in biomedical engineering, analytical chemistry, biotechnology, and sensor technology.

This book begins with an overview of biosensors, outlining their historical evolution, fundamental components, and classification. It introduces the key elements of biosensor systems, including biorecognition mechanisms, transduction processes, and signal processing approaches, while emphasizing the interplay between biological specificity and physicochemical detection methods.

Subsequent sections present the theoretical foundations of biosensors, covering static and dynamic sensor characteristics, measurement errors, and uncertainty analysis. A dedicated chapter introduces the ISO Guide to the Expression of Uncertainty in Measurement (ISO GUM), providing structured approaches to uncertainty budgeting and traceability in biosensor performance evaluation.

This book then explores the major categories of biosensors, electrochemical, optical, impedance, acoustic, and field-effect transistor (FET)-based systems, detailing their operational principles, technical characteristics, and representative applications. The discussion extends to immunosensors and nanomaterial-enhanced platforms, reflecting recent trends in sensitivity improvement, miniaturization, and real-time data acquisition.

A separate section is devoted to biomedical and healthcare applications, highlighting the use of biosensors in disease diagnostics, drug monitoring, wearable health systems, and point-of-care technologies. The integration of biosensors with artificial intelligence, Internet of Things (IoT) frameworks, and lab-on-a-chip systems is examined, emphasizing their potential in personalized and preventive medicine.

The concluding chapters discuss future trends and challenges in biosensor development, including issues of biocompatibility, stability, regulatory compliance, and data-driven analytics.

By combining theoretical rigor with practical insight, this textbook serves as an essential reference for understanding biosensors and their expanding role in modern biomedical engineering, healthcare, and analytical science.

Banja Luka, Bosnia and Herzegovina   Dr. Almir Badnjević
Sarajevo, Bosnia and Herzegovina   Lemana Spahić

Acknowledgments

The authors would like to acknowledge **Sara Deumić, MSc**, for her professional engagement in the formatting and technical finalization of this textbook. Her careful attention to detail and methodological precision contributed substantially to ensuring the quality and consistency of the final publication.

The authors further wish to acknowledge the valuable influence of their students, whose intellectual curiosity and active participation in biosensor-related courses and research activities have served as a significant source of insight and motivation during the development of this work.

Gratitude is also extended to the authors' families and colleagues for their continued support, patience, and encouragement throughout the preparation of this manuscript. Their understanding and collaboration were essential in bringing this project to completion.

Competing Interests The authors have no competing interests to declare that are relevant to the content of this manuscript.

Contents

List of Figures

List of Tables

Chapter 1
Introduction to Biosensors

This chapter lays out the foundations of biosensors. Biosensors represent one of the most profound intersections between biology and technology. From Clark's enzyme electrode to modern AI-integrated wearables, they embody the human pursuit to read the language of life in real time. Their evolution mirrors the progression of analytical science itself, from observation to automation, from detection to prediction. In the following chapter, we introduce biosensors as a concept, from their early beginnings and basic applications (Sect. 1.1) through fundamental principles (Sect. 1.2) to the quantification of uncertainty explored in Sects. 1.3 and 1.4.

1.1 Introduction to Biosensors

A **biosensor** is an analytical device that integrates a biological recognition element with a physical transducer to detect and quantify chemical or biological analytes. The International Union of Pure and Applied Chemistry (IUPAC) defines a biosensor as "a self-contained integrated device capable of providing specific quantitative or semi-quantitative analytical information using a biological recognition element retained in direct spatial contact with a transduction element."

At its core, a biosensor operates through a simple but powerful principle: a biological entity interacts with a target analyte, producing a physicochemical change that can be converted into a measurable signal [1]. The specificity arises from the **biorecognition layer**, which may consist of enzymes, antibodies, nucleic acids, aptamers, cells, or tissues. The **transducer** converts this biological response into a quantifiable electrical, optical, or mechanical signal (Fig. 1.1).

A. Badnjević, L. Spahić, *Biosensors*, Series in BioEngineering,
https://doi.org/10.1007/978-3-032-15757-7_1

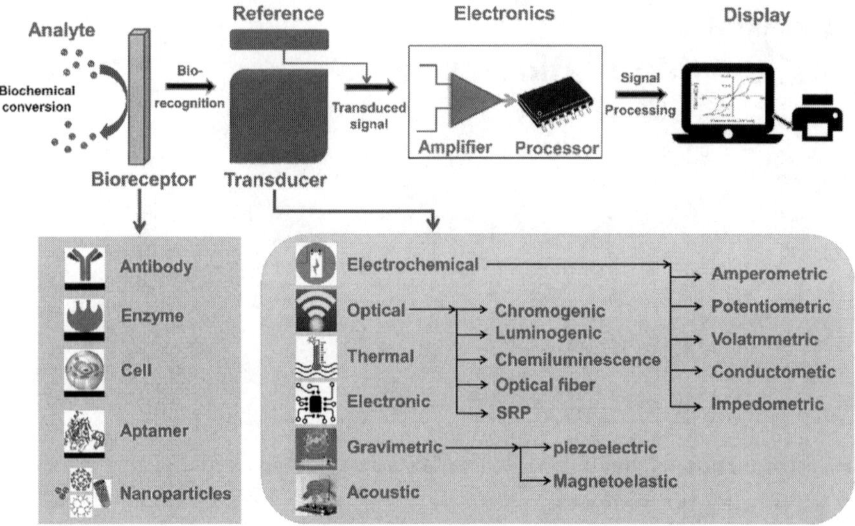

Fig. 1.1 Block diagram of a biosensor (https://commons.wikimedia.org/wiki/File:Schematic_diagram_of_typical_biosensor.webp)

Biosensors occupy a unique interdisciplinary space, uniting concepts from **biochemistry, physics, materials science, and electrical engineering**. They bridge the molecular-level recognition of biochemistry with the quantitative measurement power of analytical instrumentation. This combination makes biosensors indispensable for rapid, sensitive, and selective detection across clinical diagnostics, environmental surveillance, and biotechnology.

In contrast to conventional analytical systems (e.g., chromatography, spectrophotometry, mass spectrometry), biosensors are typically **miniaturized, portable, and capable of real-time measurements**, often without the need for extensive sample preparation. Their development reflects the growing demand for **point-of-care testing**, **wearable health monitoring**, and **continuous biochemical sensing** in diverse contexts [2].

The scope of biosensors extends beyond medical diagnostics. In the **food industry**, they are used for pathogen detection and quality control; in **environmental monitoring**, they detect pollutants such as heavy metals and pesticides; in **industrial biotechnology**, they monitor bioreactors and fermentation processes. Moreover, the recent integration of **nanotechnology, microfluidics, and artificial intelligence (AI)** has expanded biosensors' functionality from mere detectors to intelligent analytical platforms capable of autonomous decision-making and adaptive sensing (Fig. 1.2).

In this context, biosensors are no longer viewed as stand-alone devices but as **core components of integrated bioanalytical systems,** devices that not only sense but also interpret and act upon biochemical information. This transformation represents the shift from analytical biosensors to **smart biosensing systems**, which form the foundation of personalized and precision medicine.

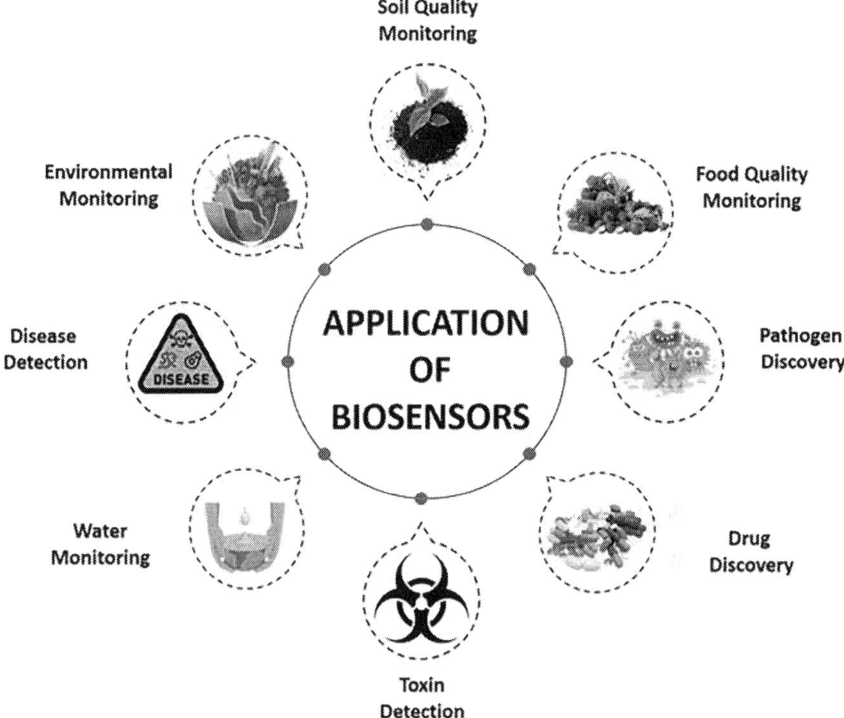

Fig. 1.2 Various applications of biosensors (https://commons.wikimedia.org/wiki/File:Various_applications_where_biosensors_have_been_used.png)

1.1.1 Historical Development of Biosensors

The conceptual roots of biosensors trace back to the late nineteenth and early twentieth centuries, when the foundations of enzymology and electrochemistry began to converge. The discovery of enzymes as biological catalysts (Eduard Buchner, 1897) and the first potentiometric measurements of biological systems provided the scientific groundwork for later developments. Early biochemical analysis was dominated by wet-lab methods such as colorimetry, titration, and spectrophotometry, which required skilled operators and offered limited sensitivity [3]. However, the recognition that biological molecules exhibit high specificity for their substrates led to the idea that **biological selectivity could be harnessed for analytical purposes**.

The notion of integrating biological recognition with physical detection matured over the 1930s–1950s, with key advances in electrode technology and in understanding enzymatic kinetics. Yet, it was not until the 1960s that the modern biosensor was born (Fig. 1.3).

The **first true biosensor** is attributed to **Leland C. Clark Jr.**, who in 1962 described the "enzyme electrode" for glucose detection. Clark, an American biochemist, combined a **platinum oxygen electrode** with an **enzyme layer (glucose**

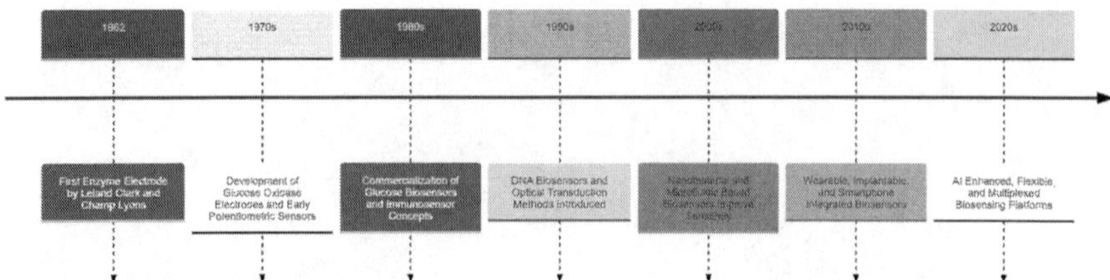

Fig. 1.3 Timeline of biosensor development

oxidase) immobilized behind a semipermeable membrane [4]. The principle was elegantly simple: glucose oxidase catalyzed the oxidation of glucose to gluconolactone, consuming oxygen in the process. The decrease in oxygen concentration was proportional to glucose concentration and measurable by the electrode (Fig. 1.4).

This pioneering device marked the beginning of **electrochemical biosensing**, establishing the key architectural principle of modern biosensors: a biological recognition layer coupled to a physicochemical transducer. Throughout the 1960s and 1970s, research expanded to new analytes and biological materials. Enzymes such as urease, lactate oxidase, and alcohol dehydrogenase were immobilized on electrodes for the specific detection of metabolites. Immobilization techniques—including adsorption, covalent bonding, and polymer entrapment, became a critical focus because they determine sensor stability and reusability [5]. The 1970s also witnessed the commercialization of glucose biosensors, initially for clinical laboratories and later for **personal blood glucose meters**, which revolutionized diabetes management.

The 1980s brought a diversification in both **biorecognition mechanisms** and **transduction principles**. The **biorecognition element** (or bio-receptor) is the defining feature of a biosensor, providing specificity toward a target molecule. It operates on the principle of **molecular recognition**, mimicking the natural selectivity observed in enzyme–substrate or antigen–antibody interactions (Table 1.1).

Each class offers advantages and limitations. Enzymes provide high catalytic turnover but limited stability. Antibodies ensure high specificity but can be expensive to produce. Aptamers are synthetically engineered, stable, and regenerable, serving as a bridge between biology and nanotechnology [6].

1.1.2   Immobilization of Biorecognition Elements

A critical design step is immobilization, ensuring that the bioreceptor remains functional while firmly attached to the transducer surface. Common immobilization methods include:

- Physical adsorption (via van der Waals or hydrophobic interactions)
- Covalent bonding (using cross-linkers such as glutaraldehyde or carbodiimides

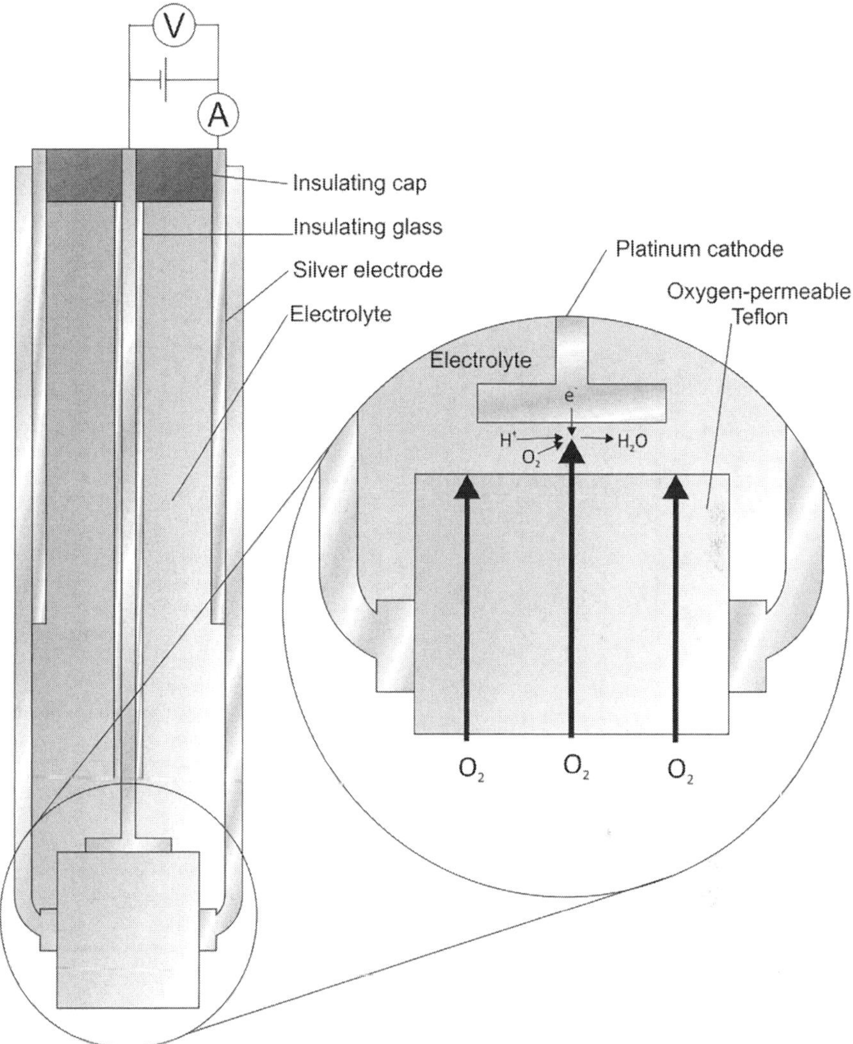

Fig.   1.4 Clark   electrode   (https://commons.wikimedia.org/wiki/File:Clark_Oxygen_ Electrode.png)

- Entrapment (within polymeric gels or sol–gel matrices)
- Affinity coupling (e.g., biotin–streptavidin systems)
- The immobilization strategy directly affects sensor sensitivity, response time, and operational stability (Fig. 1.5).

The **transducer** converts the biochemical event into a quantifiable physical signal. Depending on the underlying principle, transducers are broadly classified into electrochemical, optical, thermal, piezoelectric, or electrical types (Table 1.2).

Table 1.1 Types of biorecognition elements

Type	Biological basis	Typical targets	Example sensors
Enzymes	Catalytic proteins that convert substrates into products	Metabolites (glucose, urea, lactate)	Glucose oxidase electrode
Antibodies	High-affinity binding proteins recognizing specific antigens	Proteins, pathogens, toxins	Immunosensors
Nucleic acids/ Aptamers	Single-stranded DNA/RNA or synthetic oligonucleotides	Genetic sequences, biomarkers	DNA biosensors
Cells or tissues	Whole biological systems responding to analytes	Toxicity, hormones, metabolites	Cell-based biosensors
Molecularly imprinted polymers (MIPs)	Synthetic recognition sites complementary to analytes	Small molecules, drugs	Polymer-based biosensors

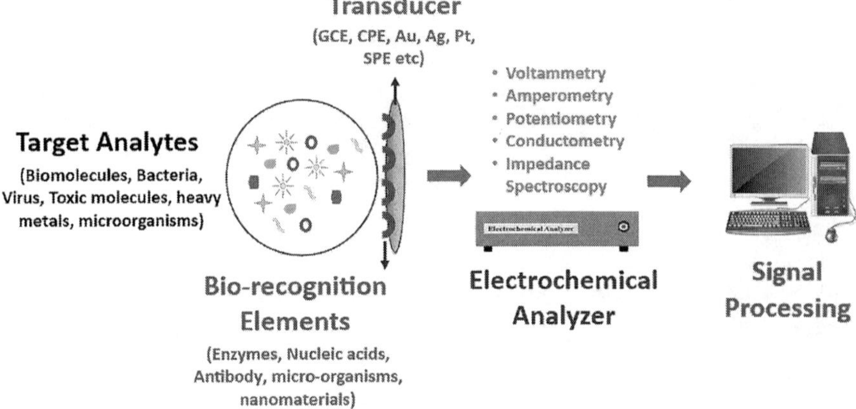

Fig. 1.5 Structural components of a biosensor (https://commons.wikimedia.org/wiki/File:A_schematic_representation_of_electrochemical_biosensor_and_its_components.jpg)

Table 1.2 Common transduction mechanisms

Transduction Type	Measurement Mode	Example
Electrochemical	Current, potential, or impedance	Glucose oxidase electrode
Optical	Absorbance, fluorescence, SPR, or interferometry	Fiber-optic immunosensor
Piezoelectric/ Acoustic	Frequency or mass change	Quartz crystal microbalance (QCM)
Thermal	Heat change due to the reaction	Calorimetric biosensor
Field-effect	Charge modulation at the semiconductor interface	Enzyme-FET or DNA-FET

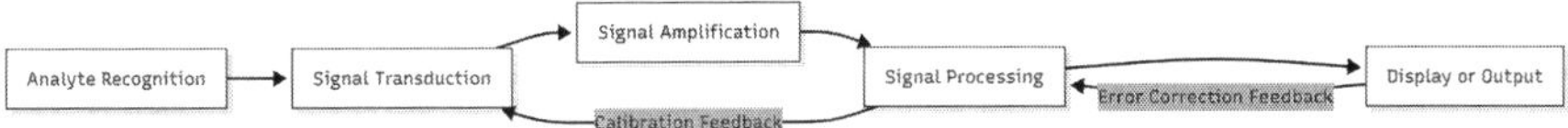

Fig. 1.6 Biosensor signal pathway

After transduction, the raw signal is typically **weak, noisy, or nonlinear**. Thus, biosensors include **electronic circuitry** for amplification, filtering, and digitization. The signal is processed through analog-to-digital conversion, then displayed on an instrument interface or transmitted wirelessly to data systems. Modern biosensors integrate **microcontrollers and embedded AI algorithms** to perform baseline correction, drift compensation, and pattern recognition. This digital processing transforms a simple sensor into a **smart biosensing platform**, capable of autonomous decision-making (Fig. 1.6).

Technologically, advances in **microelectronics and microfabrication** facilitated sensor miniaturization, integration, and mass production. The advent of **silicon-based transducers**, thin-film technologies, and microelectrode arrays enabled biosensors to enter domains that require high-throughput and multiplexed measurements [7]. The period also saw the emergence of **fiber-optic biosensors**, **acoustic wave sensors**, and **field-effect transistor-based sensors (BioFETs)**, each offering unique advantages in sensitivity and response dynamics. By the late 1990s, biosensors had become a recognized research field, supported by the growth of biotechnology, materials science, and nanofabrication.

The twenty-first century marked a paradigm shift: the convergence of **nanotechnology and biosensing**. Nanomaterials such as **gold nanoparticles, carbon nanotubes, quantum dots, and graphene** dramatically enhanced transduction sensitivity and surface immobilization efficiency. Nanoscale materials offered large surface areas, excellent electrical properties, and tunable chemical functionalities, enabling **ultrasensitive detection down to single-molecule levels**. Concurrently, **microfluidics** enabled sample miniaturization and multiplexed analysis, leading to the development of **lab-on-a-chip** biosensors that integrate sample processing, detection, and analysis within a single device [8]. Applications broadened to **environmental surveillance, food safety, biodefense, and point-of-care diagnostics**. These systems combined analytical precision with portability and user-friendliness, marking a shift from laboratory instruments to **real-world biosensing platforms**.

In the past decade, biosensors have evolved from analytical instruments to **digital health tools**. Wearable biosensors capable of continuous, non-invasive monitoring of physiological and biochemical markers, such as glucose, lactate, cortisol, and electrolytes, have become central to personalized medicine. Integration with **smartphones, cloud computing, and AI** enables real-time data analytics and adaptive feedback loops, transforming biosensors into intelligent diagnostic ecosystems. The trend toward **flexible and stretchable electronics** has further expanded their use, enabling the embedding of biosensors in textiles, skin patches, and implantable systems.

Modern biosensor research increasingly emphasizes **multi-analyte detection**, **self-powered sensors**, and **biodegradable materials** to align with the goals of sustainability and precision health [9]. Moreover, advances in **synthetic biology** and **machine learning (ML)** are facilitating the creation of adaptive biorecognition systems that evolve in response to environmental stimuli, ushering in the era of **smart biosensing networks**.

Biosensors can be classified in several complementary ways, each emphasizing a different functional or structural aspect.

Classification by Biorecognition Mechanism

- Enzyme-based biosensors—rely on catalytic conversion of analytes.
- Immunosensors—exploit antigen–antibody specificity
- DNA and aptamer biosensors—utilize sequence complementarity or aptamer folding.
- Cell-based biosensors—use whole cells responding to analytes via metabolism or signaling.
- Biomimetic sensors—synthetic systems mimicking biological recognition (e.g., MIPs) (Fig. 1.7).

Classification by Transduction Method

- Electrochemical biosensors—amperometric, potentiometric, and impedimetric.
- Optical biosensors—based on light absorption, fluorescence, SPR, or refractive index.
- Piezoelectric/acoustic biosensors—detect mass or mechanical resonance changes.
- Calorimetric biosensors—measure exothermic or endothermic reaction heat.
- Field-effect biosensors—sense charge variations on semiconductor interfaces (Fig. 1.8).

Classification by Application

- Biomedical biosensors—disease diagnostics, glucose, cholesterol, and pathogen detection.
- Environmental biosensors—pollutant, pesticide, and heavy metal monitoring.
- Food and agricultural biosensors—freshness indicators, pathogen detection.
- Industrial biosensors—fermentation, waste treatment, and process control.
- Defense and security biosensors—toxin, explosive, or biowarfare agent detection.

The quality of a biosensor is defined by several analytical performance parameters that determine its reliability and suitability for a given application. Sensitivity reflects the magnitude of response per unit change in analyte concentration. It depends on the bioreceptor's affinity, the transducer's efficiency, and the surface area [10]. Nanostructured transducers and catalytic amplification are common strategies to enhance sensitivity. Mathematically

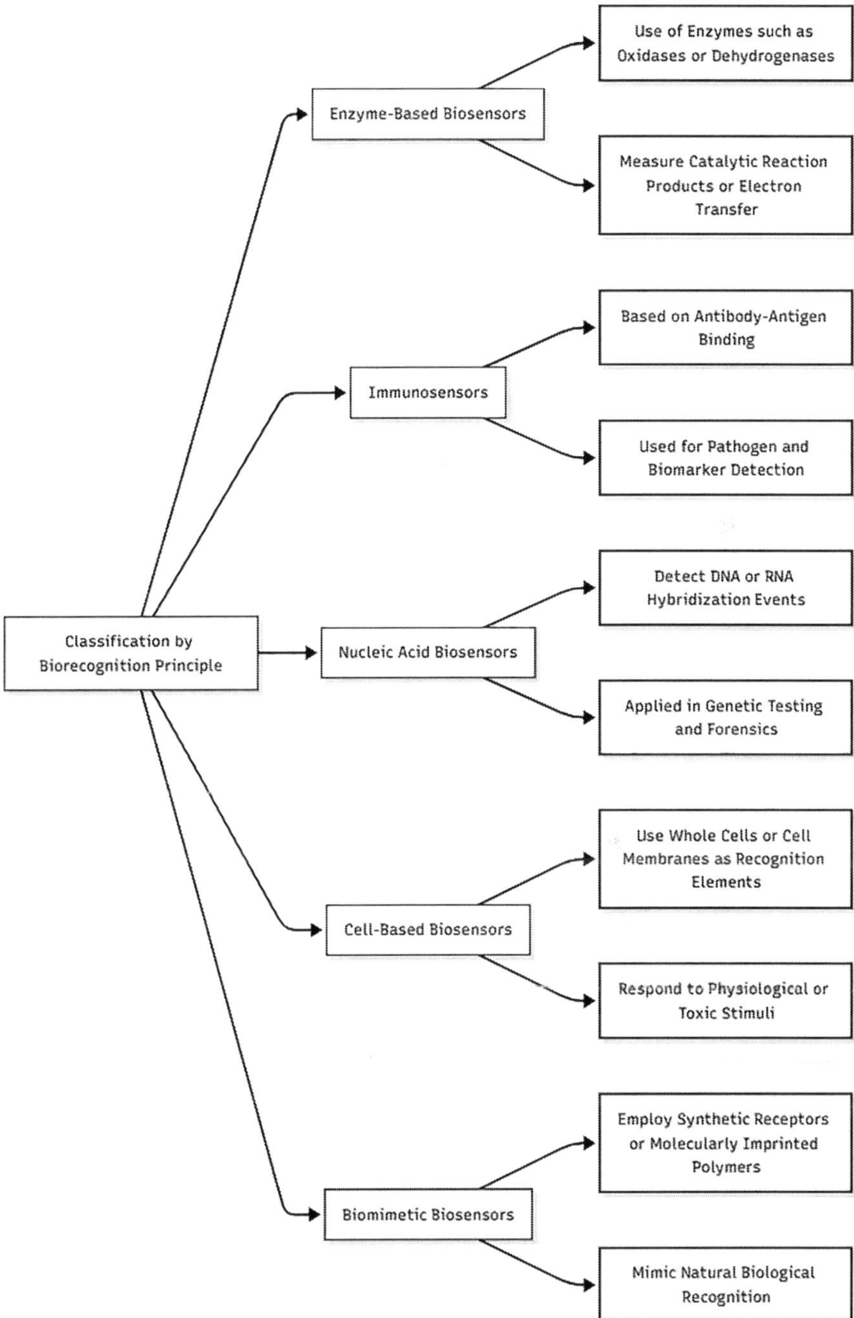

Fig. 1.7   Classification by biorecognition principle

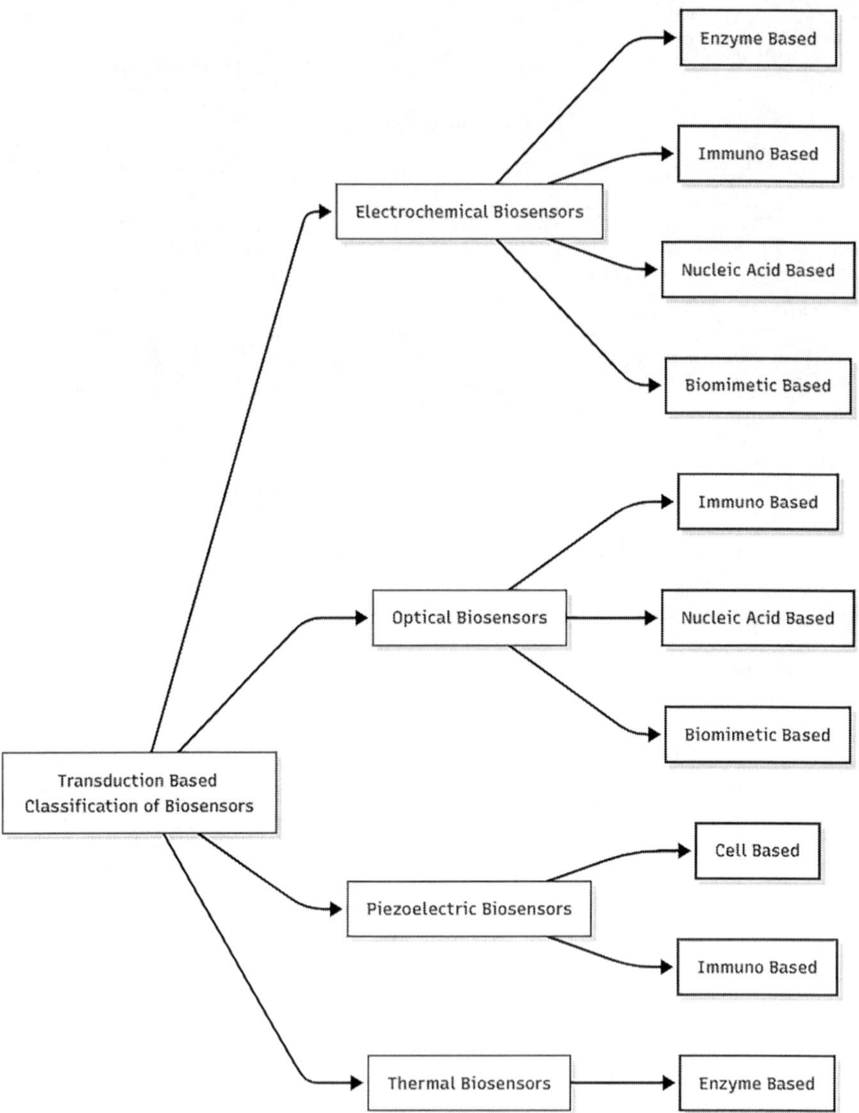

Fig. 1.8 Transduction-based classification of biosensors

$$S = \frac{\Delta Y}{\Delta C} \qquad (1.1)$$

where:

- S is sensitivity,
- Y the measured signal, and
- C the analyte concentration (Fig. 1.9).

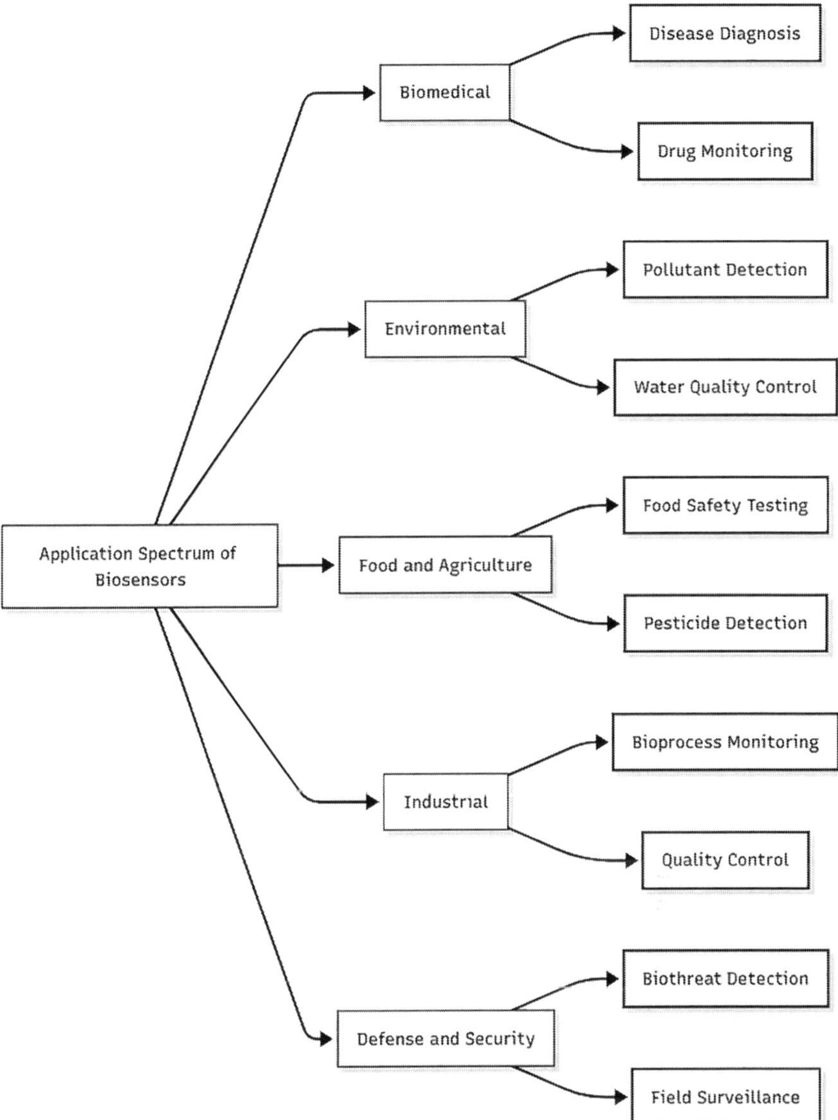

Fig. 1.9 Application spectrum of biosensors

Selectivity is the ability to distinguish the target analyte from interfering substances. Biological systems inherently possess selectivity, but cross-reactivity or non-specific adsorption can degrade performance. Techniques such as surface blocking, signal referencing, and computational discrimination enhance selectivity.

The **dynamic range** represents the concentration span over which the sensor response remains linear. Beyond this range, enzyme saturation or signal drift can

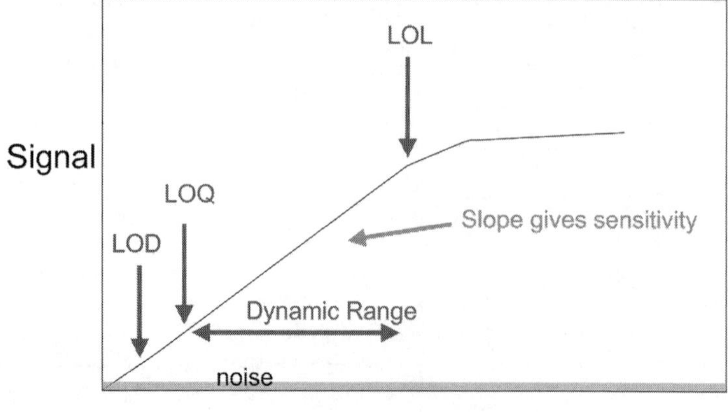

Fig. 1.10 Typical calibration curve for a biosensor (https://commons.wikimedia.org/wiki/File:Calibration_curve.png)

occur. For biomedical biosensors, maintaining linearity across physiologically relevant concentrations is essential [11].

Response time (t_{90}) is the period required for the sensor to reach 90% of its steady-state response after analyte introduction. It reflects diffusion rates, reaction kinetics, and transducer speed. Miniaturization and microfluidic integration often reduce response times from minutes to seconds (Fig. 1.10).

Reproducibility is the ability to yield consistent results under identical conditions, while **operational stability** represents sustained performance over time under repeated use or environmental stress. Stability can degrade due to enzyme denaturation, fouling, or electrode degradation. Protective coatings and robust immobilization chemistries mitigate such issues.

Limit of Detection (LOD) is the lowest concentration of analyte that produces a distinguishable signal from noise. It is typically defined as:

$$LOD = \frac{3\sigma}{S} \tag{1.2}$$

where

- σ is the standard deviation of the blank and
- S the sensitivity.

Advanced nanomaterial-based biosensors have achieved LODs in the femtomolar to attomolar range, enabling early disease detection and single-cell analyses (Table 1.3).

Developing a biosensor is not a linear exercise in assembling parts but a **creative synthesis of disciplines**. It begins with an idea, the recognition of a biochemical problem that demands a faster, smaller, or more specific solution than conventional

Table 1.3 Analytical performance parameters summary

Parameter	Definition	Typical Range/Example	Notes for Biomedical Biosensors
Sensitivity	Change in output signal per unit analyte concentration	$0.1-10\ \mu A \cdot mM^{-1} \cdot cm^{-2}$ (electrochemical); $0.001-0.1\ nm \cdot \mu M^{-1}$ (optical)	Depends on the transducer and immobilization method
Selectivity	Ability to discriminate the target analyte from interferents	$10-100\times$ higher response to target vs. interferents	Achieved via selective biorecognition (enzyme, antibody, aptamer)
Limit of detection (LOD)	Lowest measurable analyte concentration above noise	$10^{-9}-10^{-12}$ M (high-performance immunosensors); $10^{-6}-10^{-8}$ M (typical enzyme sensors)	Improves with nanomaterial enhancement and signal amplification
Linearity range	The concentration range where the response is proportional to the analyte	$10^{-9}-10^{-3}$ M	Narrow for enzyme sensors, broader for optical and FET types
Response time	Time to reach a steady-state signal after analyte exposure	$1-120$ s	Critical for real-time and wearable devices
Operational stability	Retention of sensing performance over repeated use or storage	Hours to weeks; signal loss <10–20% over test period	Affected by temperature, humidity, and bioreceptor degradation

laboratory methods can offer. From there, the process unfolds as a dialogue between biology and engineering.

In its earliest stage, the biosensor exists as a **conceptual design**, shaped by a simple question: *What needs to be measured, and why?* This question defines every subsequent technical decision [12]. For instance, a clinician interested in continuous glucose monitoring needs a sensor that operates safely inside or on the skin, resists fouling, and can function for days without recalibration. Conversely, an environmental chemist testing for pesticides in irrigation water requires a rugged, field-deployable device with rapid response but less stringent biocompatibility. Designing a biosensor thus becomes an act of **translation**, translating a biological question into measurable physics. Once the analytical target and recognition chemistry are established, engineers and materials scientists collaborate to bring the concept into physical form. In a typical laboratory, biosensor fabrication might involve **depositing microelectrodes** on a silicon or polymer substrate, **patterning channels** using photolithography, and **immobilizing biological molecules** onto these surfaces.

Each step demands compromise: immobilizing an enzyme too rigidly may destroy its catalytic activity, while attaching it too loosely may cause it to wash away during operation [13]. The art of biosensor fabrication lies in **preserving biological function within an engineered environment**. Modern fabrication techniques draw heavily from **microelectronics**. Thin-film deposition and soft lithography have enabled the miniaturization of biosensors to the micron and nanometer scale. Meanwhile, **microfluidic technologies** enable precise control of fluids in tiny channels, integrating sample preparation, reaction, and detection in a single platform, the so-called *lab-on-a-chip*.

1.1.3 From Development to Market

No biosensor is complete until its response is proven reliable. Calibration transforms the device from a prototype into an analytical instrument. In practice, this involves exposing the biosensor to known concentrations of the analyte, recording its response, and constructing a **calibration curve**. However, calibration is not merely about fitting a line through data points. It reveals the **sensor's behavioral fingerprint**, its sensitivity, linear range, and susceptibility to drift or interference. In glucose biosensors, for instance, the linear range depends on oxygen availability, since the enzyme glucose oxidase consumes oxygen during catalysis. Without careful calibration, such dependencies can produce misleading results. Analytical validation builds upon calibration, assessing **accuracy**, **precision**, **limit of detection**, and **stability** under realistic conditions [14]. In biomedical contexts, validation must adhere to strict international standards (such as ISO 15197 for glucose monitors), ensuring patient safety and device reproducibility (Table 1.4).

Few scientific devices have faced the commercialization challenges that biosensors have. While laboratory prototypes abound, only a handful, notably **the glucose test strip**, have achieved global market penetration. The reasons lie in the interplay between **cost, reliability, and regulation**.

For biosensors entering medical or environmental markets, **compliance with international standards** is mandatory. Relevant frameworks include:

- **ISO 13485**—Quality management systems for medical devices;
- **ISO 15197**—Requirements for glucose monitoring systems;
- **ISO/IEC 17025**—Testing and calibration laboratories;
- **FDA 510(k)** or **CE marking** for regulatory approval.

Commercial success requires not only technical performance but **manufacturability**. Processes such as **screen-printing electrodes on flexible substrates** and

Table 1.4 Core validation metrics for biosensors

Parameter	Definition	Typical Benchmark
Accuracy	Deviation from known concentration	$\leq 5\%$ error
Precision	Relative standard deviation	$\leq 2\%$
Linearity	R^2 value of the calibration curve	≥ 0.995
LOD	$3\sigma/S$ sensitivity criterion	Application-dependent
Drift	Change in baseline signal per hour	$<1\%$

roll-to-roll polymer production have made it feasible to produce millions of identical sensors at low cost. At the same time, regulatory frameworks such as **FDA 510(k)** and **CE marking** impose rigorous testing for safety, accuracy, and environmental impact. Commercial viability requires **reproducible mass production, cost control**, and **user-centered design**. Advances in **screen-printing, roll-to-roll processing, and polymer microfabrication** have made disposable biosensors (e.g., glucose test strips) widely accessible. If the essence of biosensor science lies in integration, its impact is measured by application [15]. Today, biosensors permeate diverse sectors, from hospital wards and food processing plants to environmental field stations and wearable health devices.

The story of biosensors is, in many ways, the story of modern medical diagnostics. Before the 1980s, blood glucose monitoring was confined to hospital laboratories. The advent of enzyme electrodes and disposable strips turned it into a home-based, minute-scale test, empowering millions of diabetic patients to manage their condition independently. Since then, the range of biomedical biosensors has expanded dramatically. Enzyme-based sensors monitor lactate in athletes, cholesterol in cardiac patients, and creatinine in renal assessment. Immunosensors detect disease biomarkers such as prostate-specific antigen (PSA) or C-reactive protein, while nucleic acid biosensors identify viral and bacterial genomes within minutes, an innovation that proved invaluable during the COVID-19 pandemic. A newer generation of wearable biosensors now blurs the boundary between diagnostics and lifestyle monitoring. Flexible devices embedded in textiles or adhesive patches track analytes such as glucose, cortisol, electrolytes, and sweat metabolites in real time, sending continuous data streams to smartphones [16]. These devices exemplify the biosensor's transformation from a static laboratory instrument into a dynamic, personalized health platform.

1.1.4   Biosensor Applications and Future Outlooks

In environmental science, biosensors serve as sentinels of ecosystem health. Traditional chemical analyses of water or soil often require centralized laboratories and time-consuming sample preparation. Biosensors, by contrast, can provide real-time, on-site data on contaminants. Enzyme inhibition assays detect heavy metals and pesticides, while microbial biosensors, engineered to produce fluorescence or bioluminescence upon exposure to toxins, act as living alarms. DNA biosensors identify pathogenic bacteria in drinking water within hours, circumventing lengthy culture procedures. Perhaps most promising are autonomous biosensing buoys that continuously monitor rivers and coastal waters, transmitting data wirelessly to environmental agencies. In such systems, biosensors evolve from analytical devices to components of distributed environmental intelligence.

In the food sector, biosensors address three perennial challenges: safety, authenticity, and quality. Immunosensors detect pathogens, such as *Salmonella* and *Listeria*, directly in raw products; enzymatic biosensors monitor fermentation processes in brewing and dairy production; and aptamer-based sensors verify the authenticity of high-value goods, such as olive oil and honey. Agricultural biosensors, meanwhile, support precision farming by measuring soil nutrients, pesticide residues, and plant hormones, enabling real-time adjustments to irrigation or fertilization. Such data-driven agriculture exemplifies how biosensors contribute to sustainability through information. In biotechnology and chemical manufacturing, biosensors serve as process-control tools, tracking metabolites, pH, and dissolved gases in bioreactors [17]. Real-time feedback enables automated optimization of growth conditions, improving yield and reducing waste. Modern industrial systems increasingly integrate biosensors with ML algorithms to predict process behavior and detect early signs of contamination, an emerging field known as intelligent bioprocessing.

Biosensors also play a critical role in biosecurity and defense. Portable immunosensors and nucleic acid devices detect biowarfare agents such as anthrax or ricin. The combination of high specificity, rapid response, and minimal sample preparation makes biosensors ideal for deployment in field operations or border surveillance. The rise of biosensors stems from their unique advantages over traditional analytical methods. They offer:

- High specificity, derived from biological recognition;
- Rapid and real-time analysis, often within seconds or minutes;
- Portability, enabling field or bedside testing;
- Low sample volume and minimal preparation;
- Potential for miniaturization and integration with digital systems.

However, every advantage comes with a limitation. Biological materials are inherently fragile; enzymes denature, antibodies lose activity, and cells perish under adverse conditions. Maintaining stability and reproducibility over time remains one of the field's central challenges. Furthermore, biosensors often suffer from matrix effects, interference from complex sample environments such as blood or wastewater. Overcoming these requires advanced surface engineering, selective membranes, or computational signal correction. Another barrier lies in commercial scalability. While thousands of biosensor concepts are published each year, only a small fraction achieve industrial adoption due to manufacturing complexity, regulatory costs, and uncertain market demand [18]. Yet, these limitations are not static; they represent research frontiers. Advances in nanomaterials, synthetic biology, and microfabrication continue to extend operational lifetimes, reduce costs, and improve analytical performance.

Biosensors are entering a new evolutionary phase, one that transcends detection and moves toward autonomous bioanalytics. Several converging trends drive this transformation. The integration of biosensors with Internet of Things (IoT) architectures enables continuous data transmission and cloud-based analytics. Biosensors embedded in wearable patches or implantable devices now communicate with smartphones and remote databases, supporting predictive healthcare models. AIanalyzes the data streams to identify patterns, enabling early diagnosis or behavioral insights [19] (Table 1.5).

Nanotechnology has transformed the sensitivity and versatility of biosensors, while synthetic biology offers programmable recognition systems, living cells or synthetic gene circuits that produce measurable outputs in response to stimuli. Together, these technologies point toward adaptive biosensors that can self-calibrate, self-heal, or evolve through feedback. Emerging research focuses on self-powered biosensors that harvest energy from biochemical reactions or body heat, eliminating the need for external batteries. In parallel, biodegradable and eco-friendly materials aim to reduce environmental impact, aligning biosensor design with the principles of green analytical chemistry. Ultimately, biosensors are moving from isolated devices toward integrated bioanalytical ecosystems, networks that sense, interpret, and respond. In hospitals, they will feed real-time biochemical data into electronic medical records. In environmental systems, they will guide autonomous remediation [20]. In industry, they will control bioprocesses through predictive feedback loops. The future of biosensing lies not merely in detecting molecules but in translating biological information into actionable knowledge.

1.2   Foundations of Biosensors

When a sensor detects a signal, the next essential step is to accurately process it. Achieving this accuracy depends on several layers of understanding: the operating principles of the sensor and the nature of the signal it produces, the characteristics of the received data, and knowledge of both the dynamic and static behavior of the sensing system.

First, a clear understanding of how a sensor operates and the type of signals it produces is necessary to ensure correct data acquisition. Selecting the appropriate hardware and software tools depends on this understanding. For instance, if the sensor generates an electrical signal, components such as analog-to-digital converters, sample-and-hold circuits, and digital-to-analog converters are required. When the signal's information lies in its frequency components, instruments capable of frequency analysis become necessary [21]. Likewise, if the measurable output involves optical or color changes, suitable spectrometric equipment should be used.

Second, it is vital to have a posteriori knowledge, information derived from empirical observation, of the signals being measured. This knowledge enables accurate data interpretation and the selection of appropriate devices and methods for measurement. Awareness of possible signal contamination or interference helps to prevent misinterpretation. For instance, a simple voltage reading may be distorted by unwanted alternating current components induced by surrounding electromagnetic fields [22]. Recognizing these interferences in advance allows appropriate filtering or shielding techniques to be applied, ensuring the measurement reflects the true value of the parameter being studied. Furthermore, understanding the response time and other performance characteristics of sensors allows for more accurate conclusions and helps minimize errors during operation.

Table 1.5 Advantages and limitations

Advantages	Limitations/Challenges
High sensitivity and specificity—Capable of detecting low analyte concentrations	Limited long-term stability—Biorecognition elements degrade over time
Rapid response and real-time monitoring	Biofouling and surface contamination reduce signal reliability
Miniaturization and portability—Suitable for point-of-care and wearable formats	Complex calibration and drift correction are often required
Low sample volume and minimal preparation	Interference from complex biological matrices (blood, saliva, etc.)
Cost-effective and reusable sensor platforms	Manufacturing cost and scalability issues for commercial production
Potential for multiplex detection of multiple analytes	Regulatory hurdles for clinical approval and market entry
Integration with IoT and smartphone technologies	Data privacy and cybersecurity concerns for connected devices

Finally, the overall behavior of a sensor can be grouped into static and dynamic characteristics. Static characteristics describe the sensor's steady-state performance after all transient effects have stabilized, whereas dynamic characteristics describe how the system behaves when subjected to time-varying signals. A proper grasp of both categories is essential for accurate mapping between a sensor's input and its output, and for ensuring that the measurement process is both reliable and interpretable.

1.2.1   Static Characteristics of Sensors

Static characteristics are features of a sensing system that can be determined when the system is in equilibrium and the measured variable is not changing with time. They provide information about the accuracy, repeatability, selectivity, and overall stability of a sensor under steady conditions [23]. The following parameters are commonly used to describe these properties.

Accuracy reflects how closely the sensor's output matches the actual value of the quantity being measured. It represents the correctness of the system's output and is often evaluated by comparing the sensor's reading to a known standard or a reference instrument with superior accuracy [24]. A highly accurate system yields results that closely correspond to the true value of the measured parameter (Fig. 1.11).

Precision describes a sensing system's ability to provide consistent results under identical conditions. It is a measure of how closely repeated measurements of the same quantity agree with one another. Precision is typically expressed through statistical parameters such as variance or standard deviation. A highly precise system will show minimal variation in readings even when the actual value remains constant [25] (Fig. 1.12).

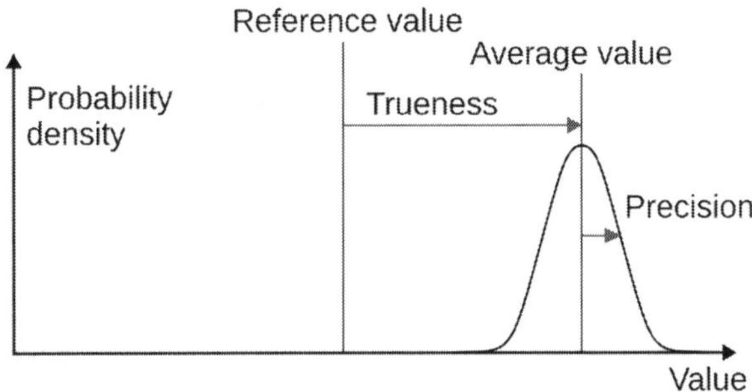

Fig.   1.11 Accuracy—trueness   and   precision   (https://commons.wikimedia.org/wiki/File:Accuracy_(trueness_and_precision).svg)

Repeatability refers to the sensor's ability to produce the same output when successive measurements are taken under the same conditions. It is closely related to precision but considers measurements taken in short-term and long-term intervals. Consistent readings over repeated trials signify a high level of repeatability.

Reproducibility assesses whether a sensor maintains consistent performance across varying conditions, such as changes in operator, laboratory, or environmental parameters. A reproducible sensing system delivers results that are comparable across slightly different experimental setups, indicating robust performance and calibration stability.

Stability indicates a sensing system's ability to maintain its accuracy and precision over time. A stable sensor delivers the same output for a constant input over an extended period, reflecting minimal drift or degradation [26]. Long-term stability is critical for measurements that require continuous monitoring.

Error is the deviation between the measured value and the true value of the quantity being observed. It can arise from internal or external factors such as calibration issues, signal interference, or environmental fluctuations. Error is often described as either absolute or relative. While absolute error retains the same units as the measurand, relative error expresses the deviation as a proportion or percentage, allowing for comparisons across different systems [27]. Errors may be systematic, arising from predictable influences—or random, resulting from unpredictable noise.

$$\text{Absolute error} = \text{Output} - \text{True value} \tag{1.3}$$

$$\text{Relative error} = \left(\text{Output} - \text{True value} \right) / \text{True value} \tag{1.4}$$

Noise refers to unwanted fluctuations in the sensor's output when the measurand remains constant. It reduces the signal's clarity and interpretability. Noise may originate from internal electronic processes or from external disturbances such as electromagnetic fields, mechanical vibrations, or temperature changes. The relationship

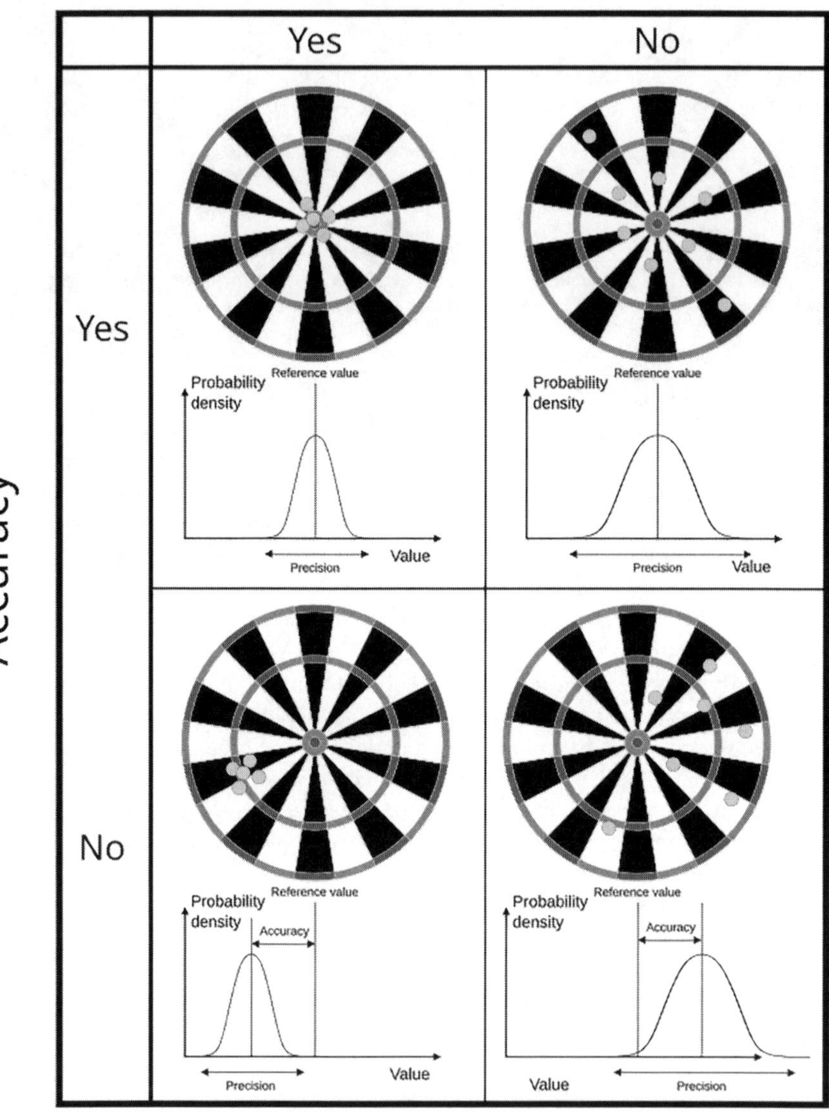

Fig. 1.12 Accuracy and precision (https://commons.wikimedia.org/wiki/File:Accuracy_and_Precision.svg)

between the signal's mean value and the noise's standard deviation defines the signal-to-noise ratio (S/N) [28].

$$\frac{S}{N} = \frac{\text{Mean value of signal}}{\text{Standard deviation of noise}} \tag{1.5}$$

A higher S/N ratio implies clearer, more reliable data. Common internal noise types include thermal noise, shot noise, and generation-recombination noise, each arising from specific physical processes.

Drift occurs when the sensor's output gradually changes even though the measurand remains constant. It represents an undesirable shift in the baseline signal that is unrelated to the measured variable. Causes of drift can include temperature instability, contamination, mechanical wear, or material degradation. Monitoring the baseline value—defined as the sensor's output in the absence of stimuli—helps quantify drift and evaluate sensor reliability over time.

Resolution, also known as discrimination, is the smallest detectable change in the input that produces a distinguishable change in the output signal. It is inherently limited by the level of noise in the system. A higher resolution allows finer distinctions between closely spaced values of the measurand.

The **minimum detectable signal (MDS)** is the smallest input that the sensing system can detect, taking noise and interference into account. When this value is measured from zero, it is often called the detection threshold. The MDS sets a practical limit on a sensor's sensitivity.

Calibration establishes the relationship between a known input (the measurand) and the sensor's output. Plotting the measured signal versus the input variable yields a calibration curve that serves as a reference for converting sensor outputs into meaningful quantitative values [29].

Sensitivity describes how much the sensor's output changes in response to a given change in input. It is defined as the ratio of the incremental change in output (Δy) to the incremental change in input (Δx). A higher sensitivity means the sensor can detect small variations in the measurand. Ideally, a sensor should maintain consistent sensitivity across its operating range and avoid saturation, where further increases in input no longer affect the output.

Linearity describes how closely the calibration curve follows a straight line. A linear sensor produces an output directly proportional to the input over its operating range. Deviations from linearity introduce errors and complicate calibration.

Selectivity expresses a sensor's ability to respond exclusively to the desired measurand without interference from other substances or conditions. A highly selective sensor can isolate the target signal even in complex or mixed environments.

Hysteresis occurs when a sensor produces different outputs for the same input, depending on whether the input is approached from above or below. This behavior introduces uncertainty and potential inaccuracies, especially in systems that require rapid or repetitive measurements.

Measurement Range

The measurement range, also known as dynamic range or span, represents the minimum and maximum values of the measurand that the sensor can accurately measure. Measurements outside this range can lead to distortions, loss of precision, or even permanent sensor damage [30]. Manufacturers usually specify this range in the sensor's technical documentation (Fig. 1.13).

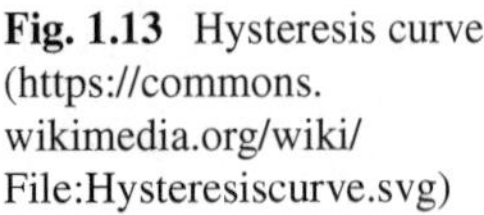

Fig. 1.13 Hysteresis curve
(https://commons.
wikimedia.org/wiki/
File:Hysteresiscurve.svg)

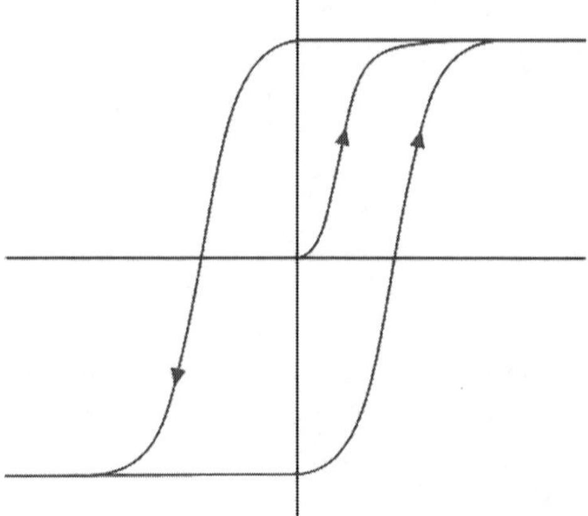

Response time is the time it takes for the sensor output to reach a stable value after a change in input, typically expressed as the time to reach a specified percentage of the final value (e.g., 95%). **Recovery time** represents the duration required for the sensor to return to its baseline value after the stimulus is removed. Together, these parameters describe how quickly and effectively a sensing system reacts to changing conditions.

1.2.2 Dynamic Characteristics of Sensors

When the measurand varies over time, the sensor's performance is governed by its **dynamic characteristics.** These describe **how the system responds to changing inputs and how closely the output reflects real-time variations in the measured quantity**. Understanding these properties is crucial for systems that operate under transient conditions, where the input signal is not constant (Fig. 1.14).

Dynamic characteristics depend on the energy-storing components within the sensing system, such as electrical inductance and capacitance, mechanical inertia, or thermal capacity. These elements determine how rapidly and smoothly a sensor can respond to variations in input. Typically, dynamic analysis begins with defining a mathematical model that expresses the relationship between input and output signals, which can then be applied to analyze system responses to different types of input functions, such as step, ramp, impulse, or sinusoidal signals.

To simplify modeling, many sensing systems are treated as **linear time-invariant (LTI) systems**. Such systems exhibit properties of superposition and **scaling**, meaning that the output resulting from multiple inputs is the sum of the individual responses, and that amplification of input produces proportional amplification of output. LTI systems are mathematically represented by differential equations relating to the input and output signals, where the coefficients define the sensor's physical parameters [31].

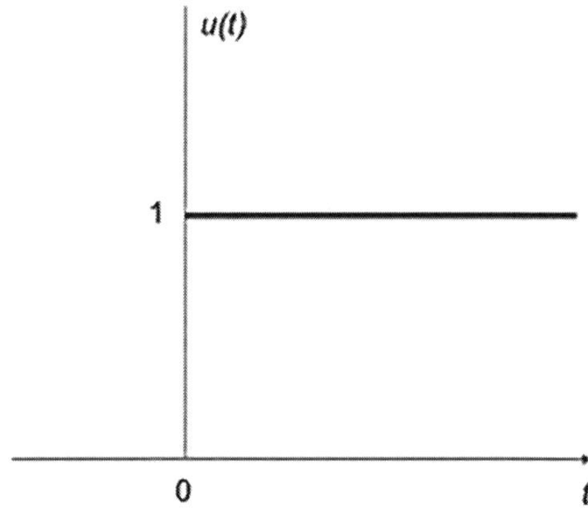

Fig. 1.14 Time variation of a step function (https://commons.wikimedia.org/wiki/File:Unit_Step_function_u%28t%29_-_SST_-_08DEC05.png)

The relationship between the input and output of any LTI sensing system can be described as:

$$a_n \frac{d^n y(t)}{dt^n} + a_{n-1} \frac{d^{n-1} y(t)}{dt^{n-1}} + \cdots + a_1 \frac{dy(t)}{dt} + a_0 y(t)$$
$$= b_m \frac{d^m x(t)}{dt^m} + b_{m-1} \frac{d^{m-1} x(t)}{dt^{m-1}} + \cdots + b_2 \frac{dx(t)}{dt} + b_1 x(t) + b_0, \tag{1.6}$$

where $x(t)$ is the measured (input signal) and $y(t)$ is the output signal, and $a_0, \ldots, a_n$, $b_0, \ldots, b_m$ are constants defined by the system's parameters. $x(t)$ can take various forms such as impulse, step, sinusoidal, or exponential functions.

When the input signal is a step change, all derivatives of $x(t)$ with respect to t are zero, and the equation is reduced to:

$$a_n \frac{d^n y(t)}{dt^n} + a_{n-1} \frac{d^{n-1} y(t)}{dt^{n-1}} + \cdots + a_1 \frac{dy(t)}{dt} + a_0 y(t) = b_1, \tag{1.7}$$

for $t \geq 0$ (b_0 is also considered zero in this case). If not zero, a baseline is added to the system response. In practice, the response of a sensing system can be categorized by its order, which reflects the system's dynamic behavior.

A **zero-order system** responds instantaneously to changes in input without delay. Its output follows the input exactly, implying no dynamic lag. In this case, the relationship between input and output can be expressed by a simple proportionality constant, often referred to as static sensitivity [32].

A perfect *zero-order system* is one in which the output shows a without-delay response to the input signal. In this case, all a_i coefficients except a_0 are zero. The equation can then be simplified to:

$$a_0 y(t) = b_1 \text{ or simply} : y(t) = K. \tag{1.8}$$

where $K = \dfrac{b_1}{a_0}$ is defined as the *static sensitivity* for a linear system (Fig. 1.15).

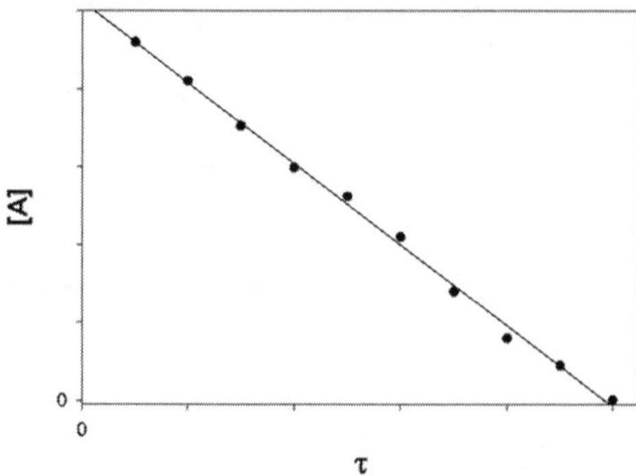

Fig. 1.15 Zero-order system (https://commons.wikimedia.org/wiki/File:Zero_order.JPG)

A **first-order system** introduces a gradual approach to the final value, where the response depends on a time constant that determines **how quickly equilibrium is reached.** Mathematically, such systems are modeled by first-order differential equations [32]. The time constant is the time required for the output to reach about **63% of its final value** after a sudden change in the input. The smaller the time constant, the faster the system responds to input variations.

An order of complexity can be introduced when the output approaches its final value gradually. Such a system is called a *first-order system.* A first-order system is mathematically described as:

$$a_1 \frac{dy(t)}{dt} + a_0 y(t) = b_1, \tag{1.9}$$

or after rearranging:

$$\frac{a_1}{a_0} \frac{dy(t)}{dt} + y(t) = \frac{b_1}{a_0}. \tag{1.10}$$

If $\tau = \dfrac{a_1}{a_0}$ is defined as the time constant, the equation will take the form of a *first-order ordinary differential equation*:

$$\tau \frac{dy(t)}{dt} + y(t) = K. \tag{1.11}$$

This equation can be solved by obtaining the *homogeneous* and *particular* solutions. Solving reveals that in response to the step function $x(t)$, $y(t)$ approaches K via an exponential rate. τ is the time required for the output value to reach approximately 63% $[(1 - 1/e^{-1}) = 0.6321]$ of its final value K. In some cases, the system response is more complex and may involve oscillations before reaching stability. These behaviors, of **second-order systems**, can be described using second-order differential equations. The dynamics of such systems are determined by parameters such as the

natural frequency and damping ratio, which influence whether the system response is overdamped, underdamped, or critically damped. A critically damped system achieves stability rapidly without oscillations, while an underdamped one exhibits oscillatory behavior [33]. Parameters such as **rise time, settling time, and overshoot** quantify the quality of such responses and are key to evaluating sensor performance. The response of a *second-order system* to a step change is shown as:

$$a_2 \frac{d^2 y(t)}{dt^2} + a_1 \frac{dy(t)}{dt} + a_0 y(t) = b_1. \tag{1.12}$$

By defining the undamped natural frequency as $\omega^2 = \dfrac{a_0}{a_2}$, and the damping ratio as $\xi = \dfrac{a_1}{2(a_0 a_2)^{1/2}}$, equation reduces to:

$$\frac{1}{\omega^2} \frac{d^2 y(t)}{dt^2} + \frac{2\xi}{\omega} \frac{dy(t)}{dt} + y(t) = K. \tag{1.13}$$

This is a standard second-order system in response to a step function for which $K = \dfrac{b_1}{a_0}$.

The damping ratio and natural frequency play key roles in the shape of the response. If $\xi = 0$, there is no damping and the output shows a constant sinusoidal oscillation with a frequency equal to the natural frequency. If ξ is relatively small, then the damping is light, and the oscillation takes a long time to vanish — *underdamped*. When $\xi = 0.707$, the system is *critically damped*. A critically damped system converges to zero faster than any other condition without any oscillation. When ξ is large, the response is *overdamped* (Fig. 1.16).

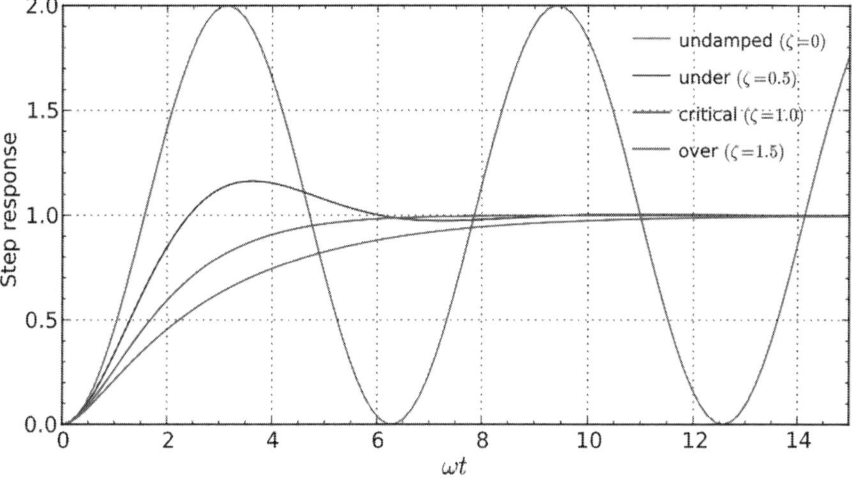

Fig. 1.16 Second-order system (https://commons.wikimedia.org/wiki/File:Second_order_transfer_function.svg)

Many sensing systems approximate first- or second-order behavior, but more complex systems may exhibit higher-order responses due to additional physical or chemical interactions. In such systems, multiple processes—such as diffusion, adsorption, or structural changes within the sensor material—can alter response dynamics, making mathematical modeling more challenging [34]. Understanding these responses is essential for designing accurate signal-processing algorithms and for interpreting time-dependent measurements effectively.

1.3 Uncertainty in Sensor Measurements

The reliability of measurement data depends primarily on measurement precision. Precision reflects how closely the obtained values correspond to the true values of the quantities being measured. The degree of precision can vary depending on the resources invested, such as the quality of the measuring instruments, the stability of environmental conditions, and the rigor of measurement procedures. Increasing precision beyond what is necessary for a specific purpose, however, leads to unnecessary expense. For this reason, measurement practice aims for an optimal level of precision, sufficient to ensure the reliability of results while avoiding excessive costs. In practical metrology, this idea is captured by the concept of measurement certainty, meaning that the results are precise enough to meet the objectives of the task at hand.

The classical understanding of measurement accuracy, first developed by Carl Gauss and later refined by generations of mathematicians and metrologists, rests on several key ideas. The **goal of measurement is to determine the true value of a quantity that ideally represents the real magnitude of the property being measured**. In practice, however, the true value cannot be known exactly. Every physical quantity in the material world has a definite magnitude, but its true value remains inaccessible to direct determination. This situation is analogous to the philosophical concept of absolute truth: it exists but can only be approached through approximation [35]. An example is the measurement of fundamental physical constants. Their values are repeatedly refined through experiments conducted by leading laboratories, and while each refinement brings them closer to the true value, the absolute value remains unknown.

Because of this, measurements rely on the conventional true value, an experimentally derived quantity sufficiently close to the true value to serve as its substitute in practice. The deviation of a measured value X from this true or conventional true value X_{tr} represents the measurement error ($\Delta X = X - X_{tr}$). Since neither the true value nor the exact error can be determined, measurement error is treated as a random variable whose properties must be estimated statistically. Any reported measurement, therefore, has meaning only when accompanied by an indication of its uncertainty or error estimate.

By applying statistical principles, an interval estimate of the error can be obtained, defining the range within which the true value lies with a specified probability P. The measurement result then takes the form of an interval bounded by confidence limits, within which the true value is expected to fall. Thus, measurements do not yield a single absolute number but rather an estimate that includes an associated level of confidence.

1.3.1 Measurement Error

Measurement errors can be categorized in several ways. One of the most common classifications is based on the **method of expression. Absolute error** is expressed in the same units as the measured quantity, while relative error represents the ratio of the absolute error to the true or measured value. **Relative error** provides a more practical comparison of accuracy between different measurement systems, since it is dimensionless. In instrument specifications, a related concept, fiducial error, is often used. It is the ratio of the absolute error to a reference or normalized scale value of the instrument [36].

A second classification depends on the **source of the error.** From this perspective, measurement errors are grouped into **instrumental, methodological, and subjective** categories. **Instrumental errors** arise from imperfections in measuring devices, such as deviations between the actual and calibrated transfer functions, electronic noise, time delays, or internal resistance. These are often subdivided into **intrinsic errors** (those occurring under normal operating conditions) and **complementary errors** (those caused by deviations from nominal conditions). **Methodological errors,** on the other hand, stem from flaws in the measurement method itself [37]. They may result from an oversimplified model of the object being measured, the use of approximate formulas, or deviations from theoretical assumptions. **Subjective errors** are caused by human factors, such as visual misreading of a scale or inconsistent interpretation of instrument indications, and are typically estimated by accounting for the operator's average reaction time and perception limits.

Finally, measurement errors can also be divided into **systematic, random, and gross errors** based on their statistical nature. **Gross errors** are large, easily recognizable deviations caused by blunders, such as incorrect readings, calculation mistakes, or equipment malfunction. These must be identified and excluded from data analysis. **Systematic errors** are those that remain constant or vary predictably between repeated measurements; they can often be reduced or corrected through calibration. Even after correction, some residual bias usually remains [38]. **Random errors,** by contrast, fluctuate unpredictably in sign and magnitude and can only be analyzed statistically. They arise from noise, environmental variations, and other uncontrollable factors. Although they cannot be eliminated, averaging over many measurements can significantly reduce their impact.

Statistical Treatment of Errors

Understanding **random error** requires familiarity with fundamental concepts of probability theory. A random variable can be described by its distribution function, which indicates the probability that the variable takes on a value less than or equal to a given number. The derivative of this function gives the probability density, whose integral over a given interval represents the probability that the variable lies within that interval.

Important statistical characteristics of a distribution include its moments. The first moment, or mean, defines the distribution's central tendency and can be interpreted as its center of gravity. The second central moment, known as the variance, quantifies the dispersion of values around the mean, while the square root of the variance is the standard deviation. The mean, median, and mode are commonly used to describe the central value of a dataset, while variance and standard deviation express its spread.

For most practical purposes, only the first two moments, the mean and the variance are used. Higher-order moments provide additional information about skewness and kurtosis but require large datasets to be estimated accurately [39]. The standard deviation is particularly important in metrology, as it directly quantifies the uncertainty associated with random measurement fluctuations.

The objective of measurement is to approximate the true value of a quantity, but since every experiment yields a finite set of results, these must be treated as a sample from a broader population of possible outcomes. The **distribution of errors** within that sample provides insight into the measurement's reliability [40]. Among all possible distributions, the **normal (Gaussian) distribution** plays a central role.

Gauss postulated that: (1) positive and negative deviations occur with equal frequency; (2) large deviations are less frequent than small ones; and (3) the arithmetic mean of many independent measurements is the most probable value of the true quantity. From these assumptions, he derived the law of error, which shows that random measurement errors follow a bell-shaped curve centered on the mean.

This distribution is symmetrical around the mean, meaning that the mean, median, and mode coincide. Its spread is determined by the standard deviation, and the probability that a measurement lies within a given range can be computed using the cumulative distribution function. Because the sum of many independent random influences tends toward normality, a principle formalized in the central limit theorem, the Gaussian law provides a remarkably accurate model for most real-world measurement data. Confidence intervals and probability estimates are therefore often based on this assumption [41].

Although the normal distribution provides an excellent approximation in most cases, it does not always accurately represent real measurement data. For certain instruments, the empirical distribution of errors deviates from the Gaussian form, prompting the need for more flexible models. A **generalized version of the normal distribution** introduces an additional parameter, F, that allows for **variation in skewness and kurtosis** [42]. Depending on the value of F, the distribution can take on symmetric or asymmetric forms, with sharper or flatter peaks.

By adjusting this parameter, experimental data with irregular error structures can be fitted more closely than with the standard normal distribution. Despite these refinements, the normal law remains the cornerstone of measurement analysis due to its mathematical simplicity and its foundational role in estimating uncertainties and confidence limits.

Several statistical distributions are routinely employed when processing measurement data [43].

- The **chi-square distribution** describes the distribution of the sum of squared standardized normal variables. It plays a key role in evaluating variances and in hypothesis testing for goodness-of-fit.
- The **Student's t-distribution,** introduced by W.S. Gosset, models the probability density of the mean when only a small number of normally distributed samples are available. It is especially important for constructing confidence intervals when the population variance is unknown.
- The **Fisher (F) distribution** applies to the ratio of two variances and is used to test the equality of dispersions between different datasets. These three distributions, normal, chi-square, and Student's t, form the statistical foundation of modern measurement uncertainty analysis.

Among all error types, **systematic errors exert the greatest influence on measurement accuracy.** They can arise from instrument imperfections, deviations in environmental or operating conditions, shortcomings in the measurement method, or operator mistakes [44]. Collectively, systematic errors associated with instruments and environmental deviations are often referred to as instrumental errors.

Formally, the measured output y can be expressed as a function of the true input x and a set of influencing parameters such as component characteristics, environmental variables, extracted energy, and time delay. The instrument's calibration function, which relates output to input under standard conditions, serves as the reference for determining measurement results. Any divergence between the real transformation function and the calibration curve introduces systematic bias. Expanding the transformation function in a Taylor series around the nominal conditions allows this bias to be expressed in terms of sensitivities to influencing quantities and their deviations.

From this relationship, several groups of systematic instrumental errors can be identified [45]:

- **Intrinsic errors**, which occur even under normal operating conditions and are primarily due to imperfections in design, manufacturing, or calibration;
- **Supplemental errors,** caused by deviations of influencing quantities such as temperature, humidity, or magnetic field from nominal values;
- **Interaction errors,** resulting from mutual influence between the measuring device and the object being measured; and
- **Dynamic errors,** which arise from the inertia of the measurement system and the finite response time of instruments when inputs vary rapidly.

Environmental factors such as temperature fluctuations, electromagnetic interference, air pressure changes, and humidity can all produce significant supplemental errors. Similarly, measurement interaction—where the instrument itself alters the object being measured, can cause measurable deviations. Dynamic errors become relevant when the input signal changes faster than the instrument can respond.

Normalization of Metrological Characteristics

When designing a measurement methodology, it is essential to select instruments that guarantee the required level of accuracy under the expected operating conditions. To ensure this, specific technical parameters, known as **metrological characteristics**, are standardized [46]. These characteristics quantify how various instrument properties contribute to measurement error and establish acceptable limits for their variation.

Normalization serves two key purposes: verifying that each instrument model meets established standards and enabling prior estimation of possible instrumental errors. Because manufacturing variations, wear, and environmental factors introduce random differences between individual instruments, allowable limits are defined statistically. Most commonly, the limits correspond to the maximum permissible deviation of systematic or random components of error.

Instruments with multiple independent sources of systematic error may specify separate allowable limits for each component, subject to the combined constraint that the overall error does not exceed the established tolerance. Sensitivity coefficients express the dependence of the measurement result on influencing factors, and their nominal values and allowable deviations are standardized [47]. When the variability of these sensitivities exceeds certain thresholds, individual calibration curves must be determined for each instrument to ensure reliable correction of systematic deviations.

Dynamic and frequency-response characteristics are likewise normalized, ensuring that instruments maintain consistent performance across their operating range. In practice, when multiple error components coexist, their combined influence may be evaluated either by arithmetic or by root-sum-square addition, as recommended by international guides on measurement uncertainty.

Systematic errors distort measurement results in a predictable way, often leading to false conclusions if left unrecognized. Eliminating or compensating for them is therefore a fundamental part of measurement science [48]. Methods for addressing systematic errors can be grouped into three categories:

- Preventive measures—removing or shielding sources of error before measurements begin, such as stabilizing temperature, reducing vibration, or calibrating instruments;
- Compensatory techniques—neutralizing errors during measurement through methods like substitution, reversal, or contraposition; and
- Correction procedures—introducing calculated adjustments after measurement to account for known systematic effects.

Preventive measures include thermal stabilization (thermostating), magnetic shielding, and vibration isolation. Calibration prior to measurement ensures the instrument operates within its nominal characteristics [49]. During measurement, contraposition and substitution techniques help cancel out consistent biases by reversing or alternating measurement conditions so that systematic effects cancel each other out.

When known systematic components cannot be prevented or compensated, corrections are applied to the measured values. A correction has the same magnitude but opposite sign as the identified systematic error. If the error is proportional to the measured quantity, it can be corrected by multiplying the result by an appropriate coefficient. Although corrections reduce bias, complete elimination of systematic error is seldom possible [50]. Residual systematic effects, called non-excluded residual systematic errors, remain and must be theoretically estimated rather than measured directly. Their combined limits can be evaluated using standard summation formulas that depend on the number of contributing components and the desired confidence level.

1.4 ISO GUM and Uncertainty Budgeting in Biosensors

In biosensor research and analytical practice, the **reliability of a measurement** result is as important as the measured value itself. When a biosensor reports a concentration, current, absorbance, or potential, that number carries meaning only when the degree of doubt surrounding it is known. This doubt, known as **measurement uncertainty,** is an inseparable component of scientific measurement [51]. Without a clear understanding of uncertainty, even the most advanced biosensing devices cannot be adequately evaluated, compared, or validated.

Biosensors, by their very nature, combine elements of biology, chemistry, physics, and electronics. Each of these components introduces potential sources of variation. Enzymatic kinetics may fluctuate with temperature, electrode sensitivity may drift over time, and sample matrices may introduce interference. The cumulative effect of these influences determines how closely a biosensor's reading approximates the true value of the measurand, the specific quantity being measured [52]. Understanding how to estimate and express this uncertainty allows researchers to communicate confidence in their results, ensure traceability, and comply with international standards governing analytical measurements.

The concept of uncertainty differs from the traditional notion of "error." Error represents the deviation of a measured value from a true or reference value. In contrast, uncertainty quantifies the range within which the true value is believed to lie. While the error of an individual measurement is unknowable, uncertainty can be systematically evaluated and expressed using standardized rules.

In biosensor development, uncertainty evaluation is critical at several stages. During calibration, it ensures that the slope and intercept of the calibration curve are statistically robust. During validation, it provides the basis for assessing analytical parameters such as precision, accuracy, linearity, and detection limits [53]. In clinical or environmental applications, the uncertainty associated with biosensor readings determines whether results meet required regulatory limits or diagnostic thresholds.

Expressing uncertainty is not a purely mathematical exercise. It is also a scientific discipline that integrates experimental design, statistical reasoning, and an understanding of physical and biological variability. By learning to evaluate uncertainty, students and practitioners of biosensor technology gain the ability to interpret data with greater confidence and to design systems that produce reliable, comparable results.

This chapter presents the principles and methods for evaluating and expressing measurement uncertainty in biosensor analysis. It follows the logical structure of the ISO GUM framework but adapts it to the context of analytical biosensing. The discussion begins with the conceptual distinction between measurement, error, and uncertainty, then introduces the two primary methods of uncertainty evaluation, Type A and Type B, followed by the combination and expansion of uncertainty values [54]. Finally, the chapter connects these principles to practical biosensor measurements and reporting practices in line with laboratory and metrological standards.

1.4.1 Concept of Measurement and Sources of Error

Measurement in biosensor analysis involves determining the value of a physical or chemical quantity, such as current, voltage, absorbance, mass change, or fluorescence intensity, that reflects the concentration or activity of a biological analyte. In any analytical system, measurement is not a single act but a process that begins with defining the quantity of interest (the measurand), proceeds through data acquisition and signal conversion, and concludes with a numerical result accompanied by an associated uncertainty.

A measurement is the process of experimentally obtaining one or more quantity values that can reasonably be attributed to a measurand. The measurand is the specific quantity intended to be measured, which must be defined clearly and completely to ensure comparability and reproducibility [55]. For example, in a biosensor designed to detect glucose, the measurand might be defined as the mass concentration of D-glucose in whole blood at 37 °C, pH 7.4. If the same biosensor were applied to a different medium, such as plasma or interstitial fluid, the measurand would change, as the physical and chemical conditions affecting enzyme activity and diffusion differ. An incomplete definition of the measurand can itself become a major source of uncertainty, as it introduces ambiguity about exactly what the sensor is quantifying.

Every measurement contains imperfections that create a difference between the measured result and the true or reference value. This difference is known as an error. In the context of biosensor measurements, sources of error arise from multiple domains: biological, chemical, physical, and instrumental [56]. **Errors are**

generally categorized as random or systematic, depending on how they affect measurement results.

Random errors arise from unpredictable fluctuations during repeated measurements. They can result from noise in the electronic circuitry, environmental variations such as temperature and humidity, or inherent biological variability of the sensing element. For instance, minor fluctuations in enzyme kinetics or in the rate of analyte diffusion can cause random variation in current output between consecutive readings [57]. These errors lead to a spread of results around a mean value, which is evaluated statistically. Random errors cannot be completely eliminated, but their influence can be reduced by increasing the number of observations or improving control over experimental conditions. The measure of dispersion caused by random effects is often characterized by a standard deviation.

Systematic errors arise from consistent, repeatable influences that cause measurements to deviate in a particular direction from the true value. They may result from incorrect calibration, electronic drift, temperature offsets, or interference from other analytes [58]. For example, if a potentiometric biosensor consistently reads 0.2 mV higher due to reference electrode aging, all subsequent measurements will inherit this bias. Systematic effects can often be recognized, quantified, and corrected. The correction may involve a mathematical adjustment, recalibration, or compensation in the signal-processing algorithm. However, the uncertainty associated with the applied correction must still be considered, since the correction value itself may be imperfectly known.

It is essential to distinguish between error and uncertainty. Error is a single value representing the deviation between a measurement and the true value. Uncertainty represents the range within which the true value is believed to lie with a stated level of confidence. In practical terms, the true value of a measurand can never be known exactly. Even when a measurement is corrected for identified systematic effects, there remains uncertainty about how closely the corrected result approximates the true value [59]. That residual doubt defines the measurement's uncertainty.

In biosensor data interpretation, confusion between these concepts can lead to misjudgment of analytical performance. A biosensor might display very small random variation (high precision) yet still yield inaccurate readings due to unrecognized systematic bias. Conversely, a measurement can have a large uncertainty while its mean value happens to closely coincide with the reference value. Understanding the interplay between error and uncertainty prevents overconfidence in numerical results and encourages critical evaluation of analytical performance [60].

Measurements in biosensors are affected by a number of influencing quantities, factors that are not the measurand but can affect the measurement outcome. Typical examples include:

- temperature and humidity in the measurement environment,
- pH and ionic strength of the sample,
- flow rate in microfluidic systems,
- electrode surface condition,

- biological reagent stability.

Influence quantities must be monitored and, where possible, controlled. When their effects cannot be eliminated, they should be included in the uncertainty analysis [61]. Each influence quantity contributes a component of uncertainty to the final measurement result, either through direct measurement variability or through uncertainty in applied corrections.

A biosensor measurement can be described by a *mathematical model* that relates the measurand to the quantities actually observed. For instance, a current output I might depend on the applied potential E, enzyme activity A, and analyte concentration C, expressed as:

$$I = f\left(E,A,C\right) \tag{1.14}$$

Such a model helps identify which variables most strongly affect the measurement and where uncertainty arises. If any of the variables are imprecisely known or subject to variation, their uncertainties propagate through the model, affecting the uncertainty of the final result.

Developing and understanding this model is therefore the foundation of a structured uncertainty evaluation. It transforms uncertainty assessment from a vague estimate into a systematic, transparent procedure, enabling biosensor data to be interpreted with scientific rigor [62].

1.4.2 *Definition and Meaning of Measurement Uncertainty*

Uncertainty represents a quantitative expression of doubt about a measurement result. It characterizes the range of values within which the true value of the measurand is believed to lie, based on the information available [63]. In biosensor analysis, uncertainty quantifies the reliability of a reported concentration, potential, or signal value and the confidence one can have in comparing it with a reference or specification limit.

Formally, uncertainty is expressed as a parameter, often a standard deviation or a multiple of it, that describes the dispersion of values that could reasonably be attributed to the measurand. It is not an imperfection in the measurement but an inherent attribute of any result derived from experimental data. Every biosensor reading, regardless of precision, carries an associated uncertainty.

The overall uncertainty of a biosensor measurement arises from numerous contributing factors [64]. These include:

- **Instrumental factors:** variations in detector sensitivity, noise in signal amplification, resolution of digital converters, and drift in electronic components.
- **Chemical and biological factors**: enzyme activity fluctuation, incomplete immobilization, degradation of biological recognition elements, or interference from coexisting analytes.

- **Environmental factors:** temperature, pH, humidity, and electromagnetic interference, all of which influence reaction kinetics and transduction efficiency.
- **Sampling factors:** heterogeneity of biological samples, sample handling errors, and matrix effects that modify the sensor response.
- **Calibration and reference data:** uncertainties associated with standard solutions, calibration slopes, and intercepts used to convert raw signals into quantitative results.

Each of these components contributes, either directly or indirectly, to the total uncertainty. Some can be quantified through repeated measurements, while others must be estimated using prior knowledge, manufacturer specifications, or professional judgment.

The **true value of a measurand** is an ideal quantity that would be obtained under perfect measurement conditions—without error or variability. In practice, the true value is unknowable. Instead, we obtain a measurement result, which is an estimate based on observed data, corrections, and models.

The uncertainty attached to this result reflects how well the measurement represents the true value. After all known systematic effects have been corrected, the result is considered the best possible estimate of the measurand's value [65]. Uncertainty then quantifies the residual doubt that remains.

It is important to recognize that even if two biosensors report identical values for the same sample, they may not necessarily measure the same true quantity unless their definitions of the measurand and associated uncertainties coincide. Uncertainty is most commonly expressed in two related forms [66]:

- **Standard uncertainty** (u): the uncertainty expressed as a standard deviation.
- **Expanded uncertainty** (U): the standard uncertainty multiplied by a coverage factor k, giving an interval that contains a large proportion of the distribution of possible values.

A standard uncertainty provides a measure of variability consistent with statistical conventions. For example, if a biosensor measurement has a standard uncertainty of ± 0.5 µA, it means that the result's standard deviation is 0.5 µA.

To report a value with a greater degree of confidence, an expanded uncertainty is used:

$$U = k \times u \tag{1.15}$$

The **coverage factor k** is typically chosen as 2, corresponding approximately to a 95% confidence level, meaning the true value of the measurand is expected to lie within $\pm U$ of the measured result in 95 out of 100 cases.

Measurement uncertainty plays a decisive role in assessing biosensor quality [67]. Several key analytical characteristics are inherently linked to uncertainty:

- **Accuracy:** the closeness of a measurement to the true value depends on both bias and uncertainty. A small uncertainty increases confidence in accuracy assessments.

- **Precision:** repeatability and reproducibility define how consistent the biosensor is under identical or varied conditions; uncertainty quantifies this variability.
- **Sensitivity and detection limit:** when the uncertainty of the baseline signal approaches the signal change produced by the analyte, detection becomes unreliable.
- **Comparability:** results obtained using different sensors, laboratories, or analytical methods can be compared meaningfully only if their associated uncertainties are known.

Uncertainty thus provides a common language for expressing confidence in results across diverse biosensor platforms and laboratories. In clinical diagnostics, for instance, reporting an analyte concentration without an accompanying uncertainty could lead to incorrect interpretation or clinical decision-making [68]. In research and manufacturing, uncertainty determines whether the biosensor meets its specified performance criteria and regulatory standards.

1.4.3   Types of Uncertainty Evaluation

When determining the uncertainty of a biosensor measurement, it is necessary to identify and quantify the various components that contribute to the total uncertainty [69]. According to international guidance, these components are divided into two main categories based on the method of evaluation:

- **Type A evaluation**—derived from statistical analysis of repeated observations.
- **Type B evaluation**—derived from other information sources such as previous data, calibration certificates, or expert judgment.

This classification does not indicate different types of uncertainty but rather different methods for assessing them. Both approaches produce values that can be treated mathematically in the same way when combined to obtain the total uncertainty.

Type A evaluation is based on statistical treatment of experimental data. It involves repeated measurements of the same quantity under the same conditions and uses the resulting variability to estimate the uncertainty [70].

Suppose a biosensor output signal is measured n times under repeatability conditions. The individual readings are denoted x_1, x_2, x_3, ..., x_n. The best estimate of the measurand is the **arithmetic mean:**

$$\bar{x} = \frac{1}{n} \sum_{i=1}^{n} x_i \tag{1.16}$$

This mean represents the most likely value of the quantity being measured based on available data.

The spread of the measured values around the mean reflects random effects that contribute to uncertainty. The **experimental variance** is given by:

$$s^2 = \frac{1}{n-1} \sum_{i=1}^{n} \left(x_i - \overline{x} \right)^2 \tag{1.17}$$

and its positive square root is the **experimental standard deviation** s, which quantifies the dispersion of the results.

Because the mean itself is calculated from multiple observations, its uncertainty decreases as the number of measurements increases. The **standard uncertainty of the mean**, denoted $u\left(\overline{x}\right)$, is calculated as:

$$u\left(\overline{x}\right) = \frac{s}{\sqrt{n}} \tag{1.18}$$

This expression shows that repeating measurements improves the reliability of the mean result, although diminishing returns occur as n becomes large.

The concept of **degrees of freedom** (denoted v) is associated with the amount of information contained in the dataset. For a simple set of repeated measurements, $v = n - 1$. Knowledge of degrees of freedom is essential when estimating the reliability of the calculated standard deviation and when later determining the effective coverage factor.

In biosensor analysis, **Type A evaluation applies whenever repeated readings are available.** Examples include repeated calibration points, multiple replicate samples, or continuous monitoring where data are collected at regular intervals under identical conditions. This evaluation captures random variations arising from instrumental noise, biological fluctuations, and environmental changes. The resulting uncertainty component provides a quantitative measure of the biosensor's repeatability.

Type B evaluation covers all uncertainty components that cannot be derived directly from repeated measurements. Instead, it relies on information from other sources, previous experiments, theoretical considerations, calibration data, or manufacturer specifications. Although less statistical in appearance, it follows the same logical principles as Type A evaluation [71].

Sources of Type B Information
Common sources include:

- Certificates of calibration for instruments or reference materials.
- Manufacturer data on sensor precision, response stability, or linearity.
- Published reference values for constants (e.g., Faraday constant, molar absorptivity).
- Historical data or expert judgment on likely variability in certain parameters.
- Specifications from environmental control systems, such as temperature accuracy.

Each of these sources provides an estimated range or limit within which the true value of a quantity is expected to lie. Regardless of how the information is obtained, it must be expressed as a standard deviation to be compatible with other uncertainty components. This conversion depends on the assumed probability distribution of possible values.

The most common assumptions are [72]:

- **Normal distribution:** used when a central value is most probable, and deviations in either direction are equally likely.

  If a manufacturer states that a quantity lies within ±a with 95% confidence, the standard uncertainty is:

$$u = \frac{a}{2} \tag{1.19}$$

for a rough estimate, or more precisely $u = a/1.96$ if the 95% interval corresponds to a normal distribution.

- **Rectangular (uniform) distribution:** used when all values within a given interval are equally likely (e.g., limited by instrument resolution). The standard uncertainty is then:

$$u = \frac{a}{\sqrt{3}} \tag{1.20}$$

where ±a represents the half-width of the possible range.

- **Triangular distribution:** applicable when values near the center of the range are more probable than those at the edges, yielding:

$$u = \frac{a}{\sqrt{6}} \tag{1.21}$$

These models are approximations but serve as practical tools for translating qualitative or interval-based information into quantitative uncertainty values.

When **calibration certificates** report an uncertainty value for an instrument or reference material, that value can be used directly after ensuring that it is expressed as a standard uncertainty. If the certificate reports an expanded uncertainty U with coverage factor k, then:

$$u = \frac{U}{k} \tag{1.22}$$

This step ensures consistency with other uncertainty components during combination.

Type B evaluation can be just as reliable as a Type A evaluation when it is based on sound information. The apparent subjectivity of expert judgment is not a weakness if it draws on verifiable experience, experimental data, and logical reasoning. In biosensor metrology, where some uncertainty components cannot be measured repeatedly, such as enzyme degradation rate or interference correction, Type B methods are indispensable.

1.4.4   Combination of Uncertainty Components

Once individual uncertainty components have been identified and quantified, through either Type A or Type B evaluation, they must be combined to obtain the overall uncertainty of the measurement result. This combination follows well-defined mathematical rules that account for how each input quantity contributes to the final result [73]. In biosensor analysis, the measured signal or calculated concentration often depends on several input quantities, such as calibration parameters, sensor response, sample volume, temperature correction, or reference electrode potential. The combined uncertainty expresses how uncertainties in these quantities propagate through the measurement model.

Most biosensor measurements can be represented by a **functional relationship:**

$$Y = f\left(X_1, X_2, \ldots, X_N\right) \tag{1.23}$$

Where Y is the measurand or output quantity (e.g., analyte concentration, current, potential), and X_1, X_2, ..., X_N—the input quantities that influence Y. Each input quantity X_i has an associated estimated value x_i and standard uncertainty $u(x_i)$. The goal is to determine the **combined standard uncertainty** of Y, denoted $u_c(Y)$, based on how variations in each X_i affect Y.

When the relationship f is continuous and the input uncertainties are small, the uncertainty in Y can be **approximated using partial derivatives** that describe the sensitivity of Y to each X_i. The general formula for the combined **standard uncertainty** is:

$$u_c\left(Y\right) = \sqrt{\sum_{i=1}^{N}\left(\frac{\partial f}{\partial X_i}\right)^2 u^2\left(x_i\right)} \tag{1.24}$$

This expression assumes that all input quantities are **uncorrelated**, meaning that a change in one does not influence the others. Each term represents the contribution of an input quantity to the overall uncertainty, weighted by its sensitivity coefficient $\frac{\partial f}{\partial X_i}$, which quantifies how strongly the measurand depends on that variable.

In some cases, two or more input quantities are not independent [74]. For example, in calibration procedures, **slope and intercept** parameters obtained from the same regression may be correlated. In such cases, covariance terms must be included:

$$u_c^2\left(Y\right) = \sum_{i=1}^{N}\left(\frac{\partial f}{\partial X_i}\right)^2 u^2\left(x_i\right) + 2\sum_{i=1}^{N-1}\sum_{j=i+1}^{N}\frac{\partial f}{\partial X_i}\frac{\partial f}{\partial X_j}u\left(x_i,x_j\right) \qquad (1.25)$$

where $u(x_i,x_j)$ is the **covariance** between X_i and X_j. In biosensor systems, correlations can arise when multiple parameters depend on the same environmental variable, such as temperature or pH. In such situations, ignoring correlations could either overestimate or underestimate total uncertainty.

If the relationship between input and output quantities is approximately linear and the influence of each input can be expressed as a **percentage contribution**, a simplified form can be used. For small relative uncertainties, the combined relative standard uncertainty of Y is given by:

$$\left(\frac{u_c\left(Y\right)}{Y}\right)^2 = \sum_{i=1}^{N}\left(\frac{u\left(x_i\right)}{x_i}\right)^2 \qquad (1.26)$$

This simplified expression is often adequate for routine biosensor analysis, particularly when input quantities are independent and contribute proportionally to the final result.

The **combined standard uncertainty** provides a one-sigma (1σ) measure of variability, corresponding to approximately 68% confidence that the true value lies within $\pm$ one standard deviation of the reported result, assuming a normal distribution. However, in biosensor applications, especially clinical, pharmaceutical, or environmental contexts—such a confidence level is often considered insufficient [75]. Decision-making generally requires a higher level of confidence, typically around 95% or 99%.

To express uncertainty in a way that covers a larger portion of the probability distribution, the **expanded uncertainty (U)** is used. This value defines an interval around the measurement result that is expected to encompass a substantial fraction of possible true values.

$$U = k \times u_c\left(Y\right) \qquad (1.27)$$

Here, U is the expanded uncertainty, $u_c(Y)$ is the combined standard uncertainty, and k is the **coverage factor**.

The coverage factor k scales the combined standard uncertainty to provide an interval with the desired level of confidence. The choice of k depends on the assumed probability distribution of measurement results and the desired coverage probability p. For measurements with normally distributed uncertainty and a large number of degrees of freedom:

Coverage probability	Approximate k value
68.3%	1
90%	1.65
95%	1.96
99%	2.58

In biosensor measurements, $k = 2$ is most commonly used, corresponding roughly to a 95% confidence level. This level is considered sufficient for most analytical and validation purposes.

When the uncertainty has been evaluated from a limited number of repeated observations, the reliability of u_c depends on the number of **degrees of freedom** v. For small sample sizes, the normal distribution assumption may not hold exactly, so the t-distribution is used instead.

The coverage factor k can then be adjusted using the appropriate value from Student's t-distribution for the desired confidence level and effective degrees of freedom. This ensures that the expanded uncertainty remains statistically valid even for limited data. In practice, when combining several uncertainty components, each with its own degrees of freedom, an **effective degree of freedom** v_{eff} is estimated using the **Welch–Satterthwaite equation**:

$$v_{\text{eff}} = \frac{u_c^4 (Y)}{\sum_{i=1}^{N} \dfrac{u_i^4 (x_i)}{v_i}} \tag{1.28}$$

This equation weights each component's influence on the total uncertainty according to its magnitude and statistical confidence. Although the expression appears complex, it can be handled easily using computational tools. Once v_{eff} is known, the corresponding k value can be selected from statistical tables for the chosen confidence level.

1.4.5   Reporting and Traceability of Measurement Results

Accurate reporting of measurement results is fundamental to scientific communication and quality assurance in biosensor analysis. The reliability of a result depends not only on the precision of the measurement but also on how transparently the result and its uncertainty are expressed. Furthermore, the *traceability* of measurements to recognized standards ensures that results are comparable across laboratories, instruments, and time [54, 70].

Every biosensor measurement should be presented in a form that conveys both the best estimate of the measurand and its associated uncertainty. According to ISO conventions, the result should be reported as:

$$Y = y \pm U \tag{1.29}$$

where:

- Y is the measurand (the quantity being measured),
- y is the measured value or estimate,
- U is the expanded uncertainty corresponding to the stated coverage factor k.

For clarity and reproducibility, the report should also specify:

- the **coverage factor** used (typically $k = 2$),
- the **confidence level** corresponding to that coverage,
- the **measurement conditions**, including temperature, buffer composition, and sample matrix, and
- the **method or model** used to derive the result.

An example of proper reporting is:

$$4.87\,\text{mA} \pm 0.10\,\text{mA}\left(k = 2, p \approx 95\%, 25^\circ\text{C}\right)$$

This presentation immediately communicates the best estimate, its uncertainty, the level of confidence, and the measurement conditions, all necessary for accurately interpreting and comparing biosensor data.

When reporting uncertainty, the number of significant figures should reflect the measurement's precision without implying greater accuracy than the measurement warrants. A practical rule is that the uncertainty should have at most **two significant digits,** and the measured value should be rounded to the same decimal place as the uncertainty.

For example:

- Correct: $0.456 \pm 0.012\,\text{mV}$
- Overstated precision: $0.4562 \pm 0.0117\,\text{mV}$

Rounding should always occur after combining uncertainties and calculating the expanded value to avoid cumulative rounding errors. Maintaining proper numerical presentation prevents misinterpretation of biosensor precision and aligns with international metrological practices.

Traceability is the property of a measurement result that enables it to be related to appropriate reference standards, usually national or international, through an unbroken chain of comparisons, each with stated uncertainties [68].

In biosensor analysis, traceability ensures that a measured quantity, such as analyte concentration, has a clear link to the corresponding SI unit (e.g., mole per liter, ampere, volt). Traceability is essential for:

- **comparability:** allowing results from different laboratories to be meaningfully compared;
- **reproducibility:** ensuring that repeated measurements under similar conditions yield consistent outcomes;
- **regulatory compliance:** fulfilling requirements of quality standards and certification bodies.

To achieve traceability, each step of the measurement process—from reference material preparation to data acquisition—must be documented and connected to a recognized calibration standard.

Creating traceable measurement chains in biosensor systems involves several stages:

Reference Materials Calibration solutions or biological standards must be traceable to certified reference materials (CRMs). For example, glucose standards used in enzymatic biosensor calibration should be traceable to SI units through a national metrology institute.

1. **Instrument calibration:**

The electrical or optical components of the biosensor—such as potentiostats, light sources, or photodiodes—must be calibrated against traceable reference instruments. The calibration certificates should state uncertainties and coverage factors.

2. **Environmental measurements:**

Temperature, humidity, and pH monitoring instruments must also be calibrated and traceable, as these parameters influence biosensor response and, in turn, measurement accuracy.

3. **Documentation:**

Every calibration, measurement, and correction step must be recorded in a traceable format, enabling any result to be reconstructed or verified later.

Without documented traceability, even the most precise biosensor measurement cannot be reliably compared or validated against external standards.

To ensure reproducibility and transparency, the uncertainty evaluation process must be documented in detail. Documentation should include:

- **Measurement model:** description of how the measurand is derived from input quantities.
- **List of input quantities:** with their estimated values, uncertainties, and evaluation types (A or B).
- **Mathematical combination:** method used to obtain combined and expanded uncertainties.
- **Assumptions and corrections:** including approximations and environmental compensation.
- **Final uncertainty statement:** with coverage factor and confidence level.

This documentation serves as the basis for an *uncertainty budget report*, which serves as an auditable record for accreditation or publication. In biosensor validation studies, such documentation demonstrates scientific rigor and compliance with international standards.

While technical details of uncertainty calculation are essential for scientists, end users—clinicians, environmental analysts, or manufacturing technicians—require uncertainty information presented in practical terms. Reports should therefore translate uncertainty into decision-oriented language, for example:

- "The measured analyte concentration is $5.0 \pm 0.2\ \mu M$ (95% confidence). The true value is expected to lie within this range."
- "The biosensor's repeatability contributes 60% of the total uncertainty; improved temperature control may reduce this."

Clear communication of uncertainty builds user confidence and promotes correct interpretation of biosensor results, particularly in diagnostic or regulatory contexts where decisions depend on measurement accuracy.

References

1. Maddipatla D, Narakathu BB, Atashbar M. Recent progress in manufacturing techniques of printed and flexible sensors: a review. Biosensors. 2020;10(12):199.
2. Song M, Lin X, Peng Z, Xu S, Jin L, Zheng X, Luo H. Materials and methods of biosensor interfaces with stability. Front Mater. 2021;7:583739.
3. Chen C, Wang J. Optical biosensors: an exhaustive and comprehensive review. Analyst. 2020;145(5):1605–28.
4. Khang A, editor. Agriculture and aquaculture applications of biosensors and bioelectronics. IGI Global; 2024.
5. Liu G, Yang Z. Insights in biosensors and biomolecular electronics 2024: novel developments, current challenges, and future perspectives. Front Bioeng Biotechnol. 2025;13:1668411.
6. Sun H, Li D, Yue X, Hong R, Yang W, Liu C, et al. A review of transition metal dichalcogenides-based biosensors. Front Bioeng Biotechnol. 2022;10:941135.
7. Raza A, Zulfiqar H, Gong Z, Chen Y, Chen Y (2024) A comprehensive review on biomedical sensors: technological advancements, applications in molecular informatics, and future trends.
8. Raza T, Qu L, Khokhar WA, Andrews B, Ali A, Tian M. Progress of wearable and flexible electrochemical biosensors with the aid of conductive nanomaterials. Front Bioeng Biotechnol. 2021;9:761020.
9. Wang S, Guan X, Sun S. Microfluidic biosensors: enabling advanced disease detection. Sensors. 2025;25(6):1936.
10. Wu Z, Qiao Z, Chen S, Fan S, Liu Y, Qi J, Lim CT. Interstitial fluid-based wearable biosensors for minimally invasive healthcare and biomedical applications. Commun Mater. 2024;5(1):33.
11. Bhatia D, Paul S, Acharjee T, Ramachairy SS. Biosensors and their widespread impact on human health. Sensors Int. 2024;5:100257.
12. Hemdan M, Ali MA, Doghish AS, Mageed SSA, Elazab IM, Khalil MM, et al. Innovations in biosensor technologies for healthcare diagnostics and therapeutic drug monitoring: applications, recent progress, and future research challenges. Sensors. 2024;24(16):5143.
13. Li Q, Gao M, Sun X, Wang X, Chu D, Cheng W, et al. All-in-one self-powered wearable biosensors systems. Mater Sci Eng R Rep. 2025;163:100934.
14. Shahid A, Nazir F, Khan MJ, Sabahat S, Naeem A. A concise overview of advancements in ultrasensitive biosensor development. Front Bioeng Biotechnol. 2023;11:1288049.
15. Zhang S. Current development on wearable biosensors towards biomedical applications. Front Bioeng Biotechnol. 2023;11:1264337.
16. Guillen-Sanz H, Checa D, Miguel-Alonso I, Bustillo A. A systematic review of wearable biosensor usage in immersive virtual reality experiences. Virtual Real. 2024;28(2):74.
17. Ghosh B, Bose A. Applications of biosensors for wound healing management. In: Applications of biosensors in healthcare. Academic Press; 2025. p. 417–38.
18. Zhang J, Chen M, Peng Y, Li S, Han D, Ren S, et al. Wearable biosensors for human fatigue diagnosis: a review. Bioeng Transl Med. 2023;8(1):e10318.
19. Ji W, Zhu J, Wu W, Wang N, Wang J, Wu J, et al. Wearable sweat biosensors refresh personalized health/medical diagnostics. Research. 2021;2021:1–14.
20. Bakri MH, Özarslan AC, Erarslan A, Elalmis YB, Ciftci F. Biomedical applications of wearable biosensors. Next Materials. 2024;3:100084.

21. Huang CW, Lin C, Nguyen MK, Hussain A, Bui XT, Ngo HH. A review of biosensor for environmental monitoring: principle, application, and corresponding achievement of sustainable development goals. Bioengineered. 2023;14(1):58–80.
22. Ogwu MC, Izah SC. Biosensors and wearable technologies for early detection and monitoring of tropical diseases. In: Technological innovations for managing tropical diseases. Cham: Springer Nature Switzerland; 2025. p. 57–81.
23. Pillai S, Upadhyay A, Sayson D, Nguyen BH, Tran SD. Advances in medical wearable biosensors: design, fabrication and materials strategies in healthcare monitoring. Molecules. 2021;27(1):165.
24. Cheng S, Gu Z, Zhou L, Hao M, An H, Song K, et al. Recent progress in intelligent wearable sensors for health monitoring and wound healing based on biofluids. Front Bioeng Biotechnol. 2021;9:765987.
25. Naresh V, Lee N. A review on biosensors and recent development of nanostructured materials-enabled biosensors. Sensors. 2021;21(4):1109.
26. Shanbhag MM, Manasa G, Mascarenhas RJ, Mondal K, Shetti NP. Fundamentals of bio-electrochemical sensing. Chem Eng J Adv. 2023;16:100516.
27. Kumari SMNS, Suryabai XT. Sensing the future—frontiers in biosensors: classifications, principles, and recent advances. ACS Omega. 2024;9(50):48918–87.
28. Bergkamp MH, Cajigas S, van IJzendoorn LJ, Prins MW. Real-time continuous monitoring of dynamic concentration profiles studied with biosensing by particle motion. Lab Chip. 2023;23(20):4600–9.
29. Chen HY, Chen C. The development, characteristics, and challenges of biosensors: the example of blood glucose meters. Chemosensors. 2025;13(8):300.
30. Muhammad W, Song J, Kim S, Ahmed F, Cho E, Lee H, Kim J. Silicon-based biosensors: a review of silicon's role in enhancing biosensing performance. Biosensors. 2025;15(2):119.
31. Pham TNL, Nguyen SH, Tran MT. Transduction methods of lectin-based biosensors in biomedical applications: a comprehensive review. Heliyon. 2024;10(19):eXXX.
32. McCann B, Tipper B, Shahbeigi S, Soleimani M, Jabbari M, Nasr Esfahani M. Perception of binding kinetics in affinity biosensors: challenges and opportunities. ACS Omega. 2025;10(5):4197–216.
33. Kulkarni MB, Ayachit NH, Aminabhavi TM. Biosensors and microfluidic biosensors: from fabrication to application. Biosensors. 2022;12(7):543.
34. Rahimnejad M, Abd Alsaheb RA, Atyia MA. Current developments in biosensors for monitoring environmental quality: a review. Environ Monit Assess. 2025;
35. Lai Z, Ouyang Z, Zhong S, Liang W, Yang X, Lin J, Li J. Dynamic characterization of optical coherence-based displacement-type weight sensor. Sensors. 2023;23(21):8911.
36. Mahajan S, Helbing D. Dynamic calibration of low-cost PM2.5 sensors using trust-based consensus mechanisms. NPJ Clim Atmos Sci. 2025;8(1):257.
37. Volosnikov AS. Adaptive measuring system with dynamic error estimation of the second-order sensor. Meas Sensors. 2021;18:100142.
38. Li X, Gu Y, Li Z, He Z, Yang P, Peng C. Three-dimensional electric field sensors: a review. Micromachines. 2025;16(7):737.
39. Li Z, Yin J, Wang G, Liang H, Zhang C, Huang M, Zhang J. Dynamic calibration of a thin-film heat-flux sensor in time and frequency domains. Sensors (Basel). 2022;22(14):5294.
40. Youssef K, Ullah A, Rezai P, Hasan A, Amirfazli A. Recent advances in biosensors for real-time monitoring of pH, temperature, and oxygen in chronic wounds. Mater Today Bio. 2023;22:100764.
41. Quesada-Gonzalez D, Merkoci A. Quantum dots for biosensing: classification and applications. Biosens Bioelectron. 2025;273:117180.
42. Harris P, Østergaard PF, Tabandeh S, Söderblom H, Kok G, van Dijk M, Iturrate-Garcia M. Measurement uncertainty evaluation for sensor network metrology. Metrology. 2025;5(1):3.
43. von Clarmann T, Compernolle S, Hase F. Truth and uncertainty: a discussion of the error concept versus the uncertainty concept. Atmos Meas Tech Discuss 2021;1–26.

44. Possolo A. Measurement uncertainty redefined. Metrologia. 2025;62(4):042101.
45. Hobbs IM, Charboneau JA, Jacobsen TL. Improving experimental design through uncertainty analysis. Metrology. 2023;3(3):246–53.
46. Kılınçer M, Özyürek M. Comparison between top-down and bottom-up approaches in the estimation of measurement uncertainty in Bisphenol A analysis by HPLC-FLD. J Chem Metrol. 2023;17(2)
47. Salicone S. New frontiers in measurement uncertainty. Metrology. 2022;2(4):495–8.
48. Moreau C, Lemesle J, Páez Margarit D, Blateyron F, Bigerelle M. Statistical analysis of measurement processes using multi-physic instruments: insights from stitched maps. Metrology. 2024;4(2):141–63.
49. Witkovský V. Characteristic function of the Tsallis q-Gaussian and its applications in measurement and metrology. Metrology. 2023;3(2):222–36.
50. Jetti HV, Salicone S. A possibilistic Kalman filter for reduction of final measurement uncertainty in presence of unknown systematic errors. Metrology. 2021;1(1):39–51.
51. Hughes F, Marschall M, Wübbeler G, Kok G, van Dijk M, Elster C. JCGM 101-compliant uncertainty evaluation using virtual experiments. Meas Sensors. 2025:101731.
52. Liu C, Duan F, Fu X, Ai S, Li J, Li T, Han P. Reducing systematic error of line-structured light sensors based on light plane correction. Opt Laser Eng. 2022;159:107217.
53. Geng Z, Tong Z, Jiang X. Geometric error measurement and compensation techniques of ultra-precision machine tools: a review. Light Adv Manuf. 2021;2(2):211–27.
54. Barbosa CRH, Sousa MC, Almeida MFL, Calili RF. Smart manufacturing and digitalization of metrology: a systematic literature review and a research agenda. Sensors. 2022;22(16):6114.
55. Leal FG, de Andrade FA, Silva GM, Freire TA, Costa MR, de Morais ET, de Oliveira EC. Measurement uncertainty and risk of false compliance assessment applied to carbon isotopic analyses in natural gas evaluation. Molecules. 2024;29(13):3065.
56. Hall BD, Koo A. Digital representation of measurement uncertainty: linking an RMO key comparison with a CIPM key comparison. Metrology. 2021;1(2):166–81.
57. Habibi N, Jalid A, Salih A, Hanane H. Estimation of parallelism measurement uncertainty using coordinate measuring machine. Int J Metrol Qual Eng. 2023;14:4.
58. Lin J, Zhang Z, Sato R, Li K, Mizutani Y, Matsukuma H, Gao RX. GUM-based measurement uncertainty analysis of a nonlinear optical angle sensor using artificial neural network. Nanomanuf Metrol. 2025;8(1):21.
59. Siontorou CG, Batzias FA. Determining sources of measurement uncertainty in environmental cell-based biosensing. IEEE Trans Instrum Meas. 2013;63(4):794–804.
60. Tallawi B, Romieu K, Favreau JO. Dynamic metrology in practice: from concepts to calibration services. Meas Sens. 2025:101642.
61. De Vicente J, Lavín Á, Holgado M, Laguna MF, Casquel R, Santamaría B, Ramírez Y. The uncertainty and limit of detection in biosensors from immunoassays. Meas Sci Technol. 2020;31(4):044004.
62. Ansermino JM, Dumont GA, Ginsburg AS. Measurement uncertainty in clinical validation studies of sensors. Sensors (Basel). 2023;23(6):2900.
63. Mustapää T, Nikander P, Hutzschenreuter D, Viitala R. Metrological challenges in collaborative sensing: applicability of digital calibration certificates. Sensors. 2020;20(17):4730.
64. Vissiere A, Krut S, Company O, Roux T, Noire P, Pierrot F. Resolution evaluation of 6-degree-of-freedom precision positioning systems: definitions and apparatus. Measurement. 2020;152:107375.
65. San Andrés L, Yang J, McGowan R. Measurements of static and dynamic load performance of a 102 mm carbon-graphite porous surface tilting-pad gas journal bearing. J Eng Gas Turbines Power. 2021;143(11):111017.
66. Monrat AA, Islam RU, Hossain MS, Andersson K. A belief rule-based flood risk assessment expert system using real-time sensor data streaming. In: 2018 IEEE conference on a local computer networks workshops (LCN workshops), vol. 2018. IEEE. p. 38–45.

67. Rayanti R, Djais AA, Masulili SLC, Wowor R. The assessment of stress indicators of mobile brigades using the periodontal parameter and cortisol titer. J Int Dent Med Res. 2022;15(3):1202–10.
68. Lavín Á, Vicente JD, Holgado M, Laguna MF, Casquel R, Santamaría B, Ramírez Y. On the determination of uncertainty and limit of detection in label-free biosensors. Sensors. 2018;18(7):2038.
69. Zhang J, Srivatsa P, Ahmadzai FH, Liu Y, Song X, Karpatne A, Johnson BN. Improving biosensor accuracy and speed using dynamic signal change and theory-guided deep learning. Biosens Bioelectron. 2024;246:115829.
70. Zhang H, Sun Z, Sun K, Liu Q, Chu W, Fu L, Lin CT. Electrochemical impedance spectroscopy-based biosensors for label-free detection of pathogens. Biosensors. 2025;15(7):443.
71. Ludolph N, Haller J, Prediger A. Measurement uncertainty analysis of single-use flow sensors. Front Bioeng Biotechnol. 2025;13:1455336.
72. Vishwakarma G, Sonpal A, Hachmann J. Metrics for benchmarking and uncertainty quantification: quality, applicability, and best practices for machine learning in chemistry. Trends Chem. 2021;3(2):146–56.
73. Ramezani G, Stiharu I, van de Ven TG, Nerguizian V. Advancement in biosensor technologies of 2D material integrated with cellulose—physical properties. Micromachines. 2023;15(1):82.
74. Mishra A, Singh PK, Chauhan N, Roy S, Tiwari A, Gupta S, Tiwari A. Emergence of integrated biosensing-enabled digital healthcare devices. Sens Diagn. 2024;3(5):718–44.
75. Rodriguez-Mozaz S, de Alda MJL, Marco MP, Barceló D. Biosensors for environmental monitoring: a global perspective. Talanta. 2005;65(2):291–7.

Chapter 2
Types of Biosensors

This chapter presents the main categories of biosensors, tracing their evolution from the earliest electrochemical devices to specialized immunosensors that define modern diagnostic practice. Section 2.1 introduces electrochemical biosensors, the foundation of contemporary biosensing, covering their historical development, operational principles, and clinical significance. Section 2.2 turns to optical biosensors, where light-based transduction enables exceptional sensitivity and versatility across research and medicine. Section 2.3 focuses on impedance biosensors, highlighting their ability to characterize cellular and molecular interactions without labels, a key advantage for real-time monitoring. Section 2.4 explores acoustic and piezoelectric biosensors, where mechanical waves serve as the interface between biological recognition and physical response. Section 2.5 examines electrical and field-effect biosensors, tracing the path from early semiconductor sensors to advanced BioFET architectures integrating nanoscale materials and wearable electronics. Finally, Section 2.6 discusses immunosensors, which merge immunochemical specificity with cutting-edge signal processing to achieve precision diagnostics. Together, these sections chart the technological and conceptual diversity that defines the biosensor field, illustrating how different transduction strategies converge toward a shared goal: transforming biological information into actionable data.

2.1 Electrochemical Biosensors

An electrochemical biosensor is an integrated, self-contained analytical device designed to provide specific quantitative or semi-quantitative data by employing a biological recognition element, often referred to as a biochemical receptor, in direct contact with an electrochemical transducer [1]. The biological element interacts selectively with the target analyte, producing a biochemical event that can be transformed into a measurable electrical signal (Fig. 2.1).

© The Author(s), under exclusive license to Springer Nature Switzerland AG 2026

A. Badnjević, L. Spahić, *Biosensors*, Series in BioEngineering, https://doi.org/10.1007/978-3-032-15757-7_2

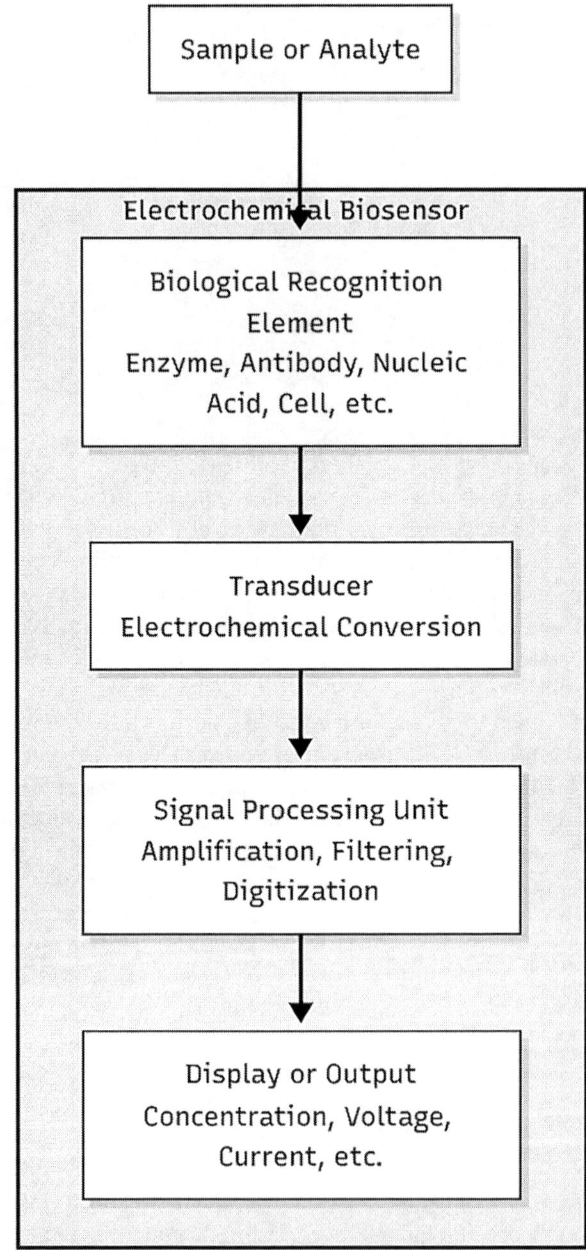

Fig. 2.1 General architecture of an electrochemical biosensor

Unlike conventional bioanalytical systems that require repetitive reagent additions or complex processing steps, electrochemical biosensors can be repeatedly calibrated and used directly. This property makes them distinct from broader analytical assays that rely on external reagent-based reactions. In some cases, biosensors are intended for single use, particularly when sterility, contamination control, or sample integrity is a concern [2]. These single-use systems, often designed for rapid and reproducible operation, are referred to as disposable biosensors and are ideal for applications where continuous monitoring is unnecessary or impractical.

Biosensors can be categorized according to two primary principles: the mechanism that provides biological specificity and the physicochemical mode of signal transduction. The biological recognition element may rely on catalytic reactions, most commonly enzyme-mediated, or on equilibrium-based binding reactions involving macromolecules such as antibodies, nucleic acids, or receptors. These macromolecules can be naturally derived, genetically engineered, or synthetically produced, depending on the application [3]. In equilibrium-based sensors, the analyte interacts with the immobilized biocomplexing agent without further consumption, allowing steady-state measurements over time (Table 2.1).

From a functional standpoint, electrochemical biosensors are also recognized as part of the "Point-of-Care" (POC) category of diagnostic devices. POC biosensors are characterized by their portability, speed, and ease of use, making them suitable for bedside testing, fieldwork, and on-site diagnostics. Another way to classify biosensors is based on the type of analytes or reactions they detect. Some are designed for direct monitoring, in which the analyte concentration is measured, while others perform indirect monitoring, detecting substances that act as inhibitors or activators of the biological recognition element. This dual capability extends the range of biosensor applications across clinical diagnostics, food safety, and environmental testing.

The rapid development and diversification of biosensor technology have created challenges in maintaining uniform performance definitions. As a result, organizations such as the International Union of Pure and Applied Chemistry (IUPAC) recommend standardized performance criteria to ensure clarity and reproducibility in biosensor evaluation. These criteria encompass calibration parameters—including sensitivity, operating range, linearity, detection and quantification limits—as well as selectivity, stability, response and recovery times, sample flow characteristics, repeatability, and shelf life [4]. Establishing consistent terminology and

Table 2.1 Classification of biosensors by recognition mechanism and transduction principle

Basis of classification	Category	Example biological element	Example transducer	Typical analyte
Catalytic	Enzyme-based	Glucose oxidase	Amperometric	Glucose
Affinity	Antibody-based	Immunoglobulin G	Potentiometric	Pathogen antigen
Nucleic-acid	DNA probe	Conductometric	DNA mutation	
Cell-based	Whole cell	Impedimetric	Toxin detection	

performance standards helps researchers, manufacturers, and regulatory bodies compare and validate biosensor technologies.

Electrochemical biosensors uniquely combine the high sensitivity of electroanalytical methods with the intrinsic bioselectivity of biological recognition elements. In operation, the biological component interacts with its target analyte, generating a catalytic or binding event that is converted into an electrical signal by the transducer. The output signal is directly or indirectly proportional to the analyte concentration, enabling precise quantification. These sensors have advanced from laboratory prototypes to commercially available products widely applied in clinical diagnostics, environmental monitoring, agriculture, and industry. Their evolution into routine use underscores the success of integrating biochemical recognition with electrochemical detection. Electrochemical biosensors can generally be grouped into two main categories: biocatalytic sensors, which utilize enzyme-mediated reactions, and affinity sensors, which depend on molecular binding interactions. Among all detection strategies, electrochemical biosensors have gained substantial popularity for detecting a broad range of diseases and analytes. Their advantages include short detection time, simple instrumentation, affordability, and portability, making them ideal for use in POC diagnostic platforms. Within this framework, several electrochemical configurations have been developed, such as voltammetric and amperometric biosensors, impedimetric biosensors, potentiometric biosensors, and field-effect transistor (FET)-based biosensors. These platforms collectively illustrate the versatility and practical value of electrochemical sensing in modern diagnostics.

2.1.1   History

Over the past five decades, the term biosensor has appeared frequently in scientific literature, reflecting the field's growing interdisciplinary appeal. Researchers from various backgrounds, including chemistry, physics, microbiology, materials science, and electrical engineering, have each contributed to different aspects of biosensor design and application. From these diverse perspectives, it becomes evident that the concept of a biosensor has evolved significantly over time.

In the early years of this field, approximately 50 years ago, the term "biosensor" was often used rather broadly. At that stage, some researchers described it simply as a self-contained analytical device capable of detecting the concentration of a chemical species in a biological sample. This early description, however, lacked precision, as it did not explicitly include a biologically active component as an integral part of the device [5, 6]. As a result, even physical instruments such as thermometers and chemical sensors, including microelectrodes implanted into biological tissues, were sometimes mistakenly categorized as biosensors.

As understanding progressed, the definition became more refined. A biosensor is now recognized as a device that combines a biological sensing material—commonly referred to as a molecular biological recognition element, with a physical or chemical transducer. This configuration enables the translation of biochemical interactions into measurable electrical signals. More recently, advances in materials science and synthetic chemistry have broadened this definition further to include systems in which biological materials are replaced or mimicked by synthetic compounds that replicate natural recognition functions (Fig. 2.2).

The origins of electrochemical biosensors can be traced back to the work of Professor Leland C. Clark in the 1950s. In 1956, he developed an oxygen electrode that later inspired the first practical enzyme-based biosensor. By 1962, during a symposium at the New York Academy of Sciences, Clark presented the concept of enhancing conventional electrochemical sensors, such as pH, potentiometric, and conductometric devices—by integrating enzymatic transducers into a sealed membrane assembly. His pioneering work demonstrated that coupling glucose oxidase to an oxygen electrode produced a measurable decrease in oxygen concentration, directly proportional to glucose concentration [7]. This innovation, described as an "enzyme electrode," laid the foundation for modern biosensors.

Following Clark's breakthrough, additional progress was made when Updike and Hicks in 1967 used a similar approach, immobilizing glucose oxidase within a polyacrylamide gel on the surface of an oxygen electrode to enable rapid, quantitative glucose measurements. Around the same time, other researchers explored alternative detection methods. In 1969, Guilbault and Montalvo developed a urea sensor by coupling urease with glass electrodes to enable potentiometric measurements. By the early 1970s, several studies confirmed the feasibility of combining enzymes with electrochemical transducers, leading to a rapid expansion of biosensor research.

During this early period, the concept of a biosensor was considered novel, as it brought together biological components and electrochemical devices in unprecedented ways. Within the electrochemical community, interest in ion-selective electrodes (ISEs) was already strong, and many of the principles used in ISE development were naturally extended to biosensors. Researchers soon recognized that by coupling biological materials to electrochemical sensors, it was possible to detect compounds that were neither electroactive nor ionic, such as glucose and other biomolecules. This realization opened a new dimension for analytical chemistry. Consequently, laboratories focused on ISE development became pioneers in electroanalytical biosensor research.

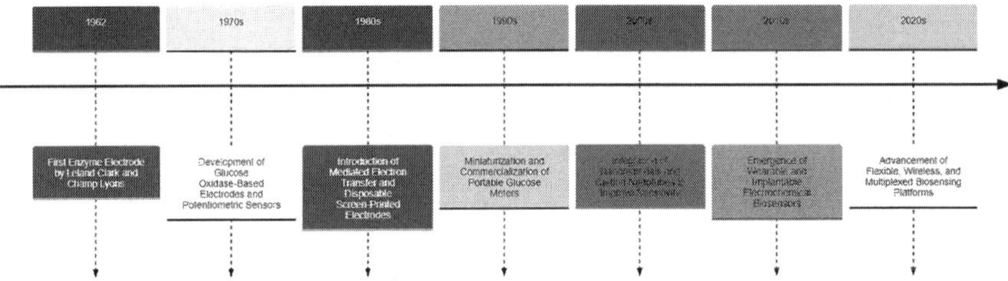

Fig. 2.2 Timeline of key developments in electrochemical biosensors

One of the earliest examples of this interdisciplinary approach was the work of Professor G. Rechnitz, who designed a biosensor to detect amygdalin by coupling a cyanide-selective electrode with the enzyme β-glucosidase. This combination produced benzaldehyde and cyanide as measurable products, illustrating the versatility of enzyme-transducer systems [8]. From there, researchers began systematically varying both the biological elements, ranging from single enzymes to complex biological matrices, and the types of transducers, including potentiometric, amperometric, optical, thermometric, and later piezoelectric and magnetic devices.

As biosensor technology diversified, two primary categories emerged based on the type of biorecognition mechanism: catalytic elements, which rely on enzyme activity or metabolic reactions within cells and tissues, and affinity elements, which depend on selective binding interactions involving antibodies, lectins, nucleic acids, and synthetic ligands. Together, these categories define the fundamental basis of biomolecular sensing.

Biomolecular sensing encompasses the detection of analytes of biological significance, ranging from small metabolites to macromolecules of environmental, clinical, or industrial importance. The ability to exploit the selectivity of biological elements for precise analyte recognition has been the main driving force behind biosensor innovation. As research advanced, biosensors became indispensable analytical tools across multiple domains, offering a combination of specificity, sensitivity, and real-time measurement capabilities that traditional methods often could not achieve.

2.1.2 Technical Characteristics

Detection techniques are among the most critical components in the development of **point-of-care (POC) diagnostic systems** because they directly determine a device's efficiency, sensitivity, and overall accuracy. The creation of effective biosensors for POC diagnostics, therefore, depends heavily on the development of novel detection methods capable of providing rapid, highly sensitive analysis of infectious and metabolic diseases. These detection strategies include electrochemical, fluorescence-based, surface-enhanced Raman scattering (SERS), colorimetric, surface plasmon resonance (SPR), and magnetic biosensors. Each of these platforms offers unique advantages depending on the target analyte and the intended operating environment.

To ensure that biosensors can be used reliably by non-specialists, certain design criteria must be met. First, the biological catalyst or recognition element must exhibit high specificity toward the intended analyte, maintain stability under normal storage and operating conditions, and show minimal variability between assays. Second, the biochemical reaction should be largely independent of external physical parameters such as temperature, pH, and stirring rate, allowing the sensor to analyze samples with minimal pre-treatment. When cofactors or coenzymes are required for enzymatic activity, they should ideally be co-immobilized with the enzyme to prevent losses that could affect reproducibility [9]. Third, the biosensor's response

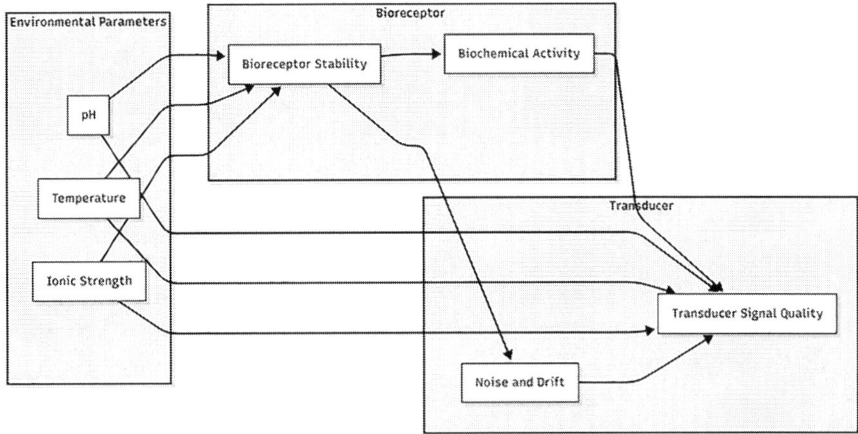

Fig. 2.3 Design requirements and influencing factors diagram

should be accurate, precise, and reproducible, maintaining linearity across the desired concentration range while being resistant to electrical noise and other forms of signal interference generated by the transducer (Fig. 2.3).

In clinical or biomedical applications where invasive monitoring is necessary, the biosensor probe must be miniaturized and biocompatible, causing no toxic or immunogenic effects. It should remain resistant to inactivation or enzymatic degradation under physiological conditions. Furthermore, for rapid or real-time monitoring of analytes in human samples, the biosensor must provide continuous or near-instantaneous readings. From an engineering perspective, the complete device should be inexpensive, compact, portable, and operable by individuals with minimal technical training.

The selectivity of biosensors arises from the ability to engineer specific molecular interactions by immobilizing biological recognition elements on the transducer surface. These elements, such as enzymes, nucleic acids, antibodies, cells, and receptors, bind selectively to their respective targets. Among them, enzymes are particularly common due to their catalytic efficiency and substrate specificity. However, for biosensors to fully exploit this selective interaction, the sensor's surface architecture must simultaneously minimize nonspecific binding and environmental interference.

Considerable research efforts have been devoted to improving the long-term stability and selectivity of sensor surfaces, especially for applications in biological fluids that contain numerous potentially interfering substances. Investigations into advanced surface modifications have led to the development of functional coatings that preserve the activity of immobilized biocomponents while resisting fouling and degradation over extended periods [10].

Today, biosensors have become standard instruments in laboratories worldwide, with an increasing number finding practical application in diagnostic testing. Despite this progress, the widespread commercialization of low-cost, handheld biosensors remains limited, with glucose meters serving as the most prominent success story. The main barriers to broader adoption of POC biosensors include the difficulty of miniaturizing certain transduction principles, ensuring consistent mass production, and achieving cost-effective fabrication at scale. As a result, many sophisticated biosensing technologies still require specialized laboratories and trained personnel, restricting their use outside controlled environments.

Electrochemical biosensors, in particular, have faced challenges related to achieving sufficiently high sensitivity and signal specificity in complex biological samples. Variations in pH, ionic strength, and matrix composition can significantly affect sensor performance, especially in immunosensors and affinity-based systems [11]. However, continual technological advancements are addressing these issues, including the incorporation of multiple enzyme labels to amplify signal intensity and the integration of nanostructured materials that enhance electron transfer efficiency.

The merging of expertise from fields such as biochemistry, electrochemistry, solid-state physics, bioengineering, and materials science has paved the way for a new generation of biosensors. These next-generation devices combine high selectivity, sensitivity, and stability with miniaturized architectures and advanced data processing capabilities. The integration of microelectronics and surface engineering enables researchers to produce reliable micro- and nanoscale biosensors and sensor arrays. Such systems promise faster response times, greater accuracy, and enhanced multiplexing capabilities, marking a significant step toward highly specific and cost-efficient analytical technologies suitable for both laboratory and point-of-care environments.

Hardware

Electrochemical biosensors are among the most frequently used devices in point-of-care diagnostics because they can efficiently convert biological signals into measurable electrical responses. This process is achieved through an electrochemical transducer, typically composed of one or more electrodes. These sensors combine biological recognition elements with electronic components to detect specific analytes in complex biological fluids such as blood, saliva, or sweat. The result is a system that offers rapid signal readouts, high sensitivity, and the potential for miniaturization, enabling integration into portable or wearable diagnostic platforms for real-time monitoring, such as home-use glucose meters.

Every electrochemical biosensor contains a few essential components that work in unison to translate a biochemical event into an electrical output [12]:

- **Working electrode:** This is the primary site where the biochemical interaction occurs. It hosts the immobilized biological recognition element, such as an enzyme, antibody, or nucleic acid, and serves as the surface where analyte recognition or catalysis generates an electrochemical signal. The working electrode's composition and surface characteristics largely determine the sensor's sensitivity and specificity.
- **Reference electrode:** The reference electrode maintains a constant and well-defined potential, providing a stable reference point for measuring the potential

of the working electrode. Its role ensures accurate and reproducible readings independent of variations in current flow.

- **Counter (auxiliary) electrode:** This electrode completes the circuit by allowing current to flow through the system. It balances the current generated at the working electrode to maintain electrochemical stability during measurements.
- **Bioreceptors:** These are biologically derived molecules, such as enzymes, antibodies, nucleic acids, or whole cells, that selectively interact with the target analyte. Their specificity forms the foundation of the biosensor's ability to distinguish the desired analyte from other substances present in a sample.
- **Electronic transducer:** This component translates the biochemical interaction into an electrical signal. It also facilitates the immobilization of biomolecules and supports electron transfer between the biological element and the electrode surface.
- **Signal amplifier, processor, and display system:** The generated electrical signal is often too weak for direct measurement, so it must be amplified and processed. The processed signal is then converted into a readable format, typically a numerical value or a graphical display, representing the analyte concentration.

Collectively, these components form a functional chain that begins with molecular recognition and culminates in a quantifiable digital output. Advances in microfabrication and materials engineering have significantly improved the performance of these elements, leading to smaller, faster, and more reliable biosensors (Fig. 2.4).

Continuous improvements in hardware design have made modern electrochemical biosensors increasingly versatile and user-friendly. Many current devices integrate multiple electrodes into compact platforms, employ nanostructured materials to enhance sensitivity, and use wireless interfaces for data transfer. These innovations have transformed electrochemical biosensors into practical diagnostic tools, enabling efficient health monitoring, environmental testing, and biochemical analysis without the need for large laboratory setups (Table 2.2).

Thanks to ongoing technological advancements, biosensors have evolved into essential diagnostic instruments that assist users across healthcare, research, and industry. Their integration with modern microelectronics, flexible substrates, and portable interfaces continues to enhance accessibility, precision, and reliability— making them indispensable for everyday biomedical applications.

Software

The software used in electrochemical biosensing plays a crucial role in controlling measurements, processing data, and ensuring accurate interpretation of electrochemical reactions. Among the most important tools in this context are **potentiostats and galvanostats,** which serve as the core instruments for regulating voltage and current during electrochemical experiments [13]. These devices are indispensable for research, development, and quality control in electrochemistry, corrosion analysis, fuel cell testing, and battery evaluation.

A galvanostat operates by controlling the current flowing through the electrochemical cell while monitoring the resulting potential changes. In contrast, a potentiostat maintains a fixed potential between the working and reference electrodes and

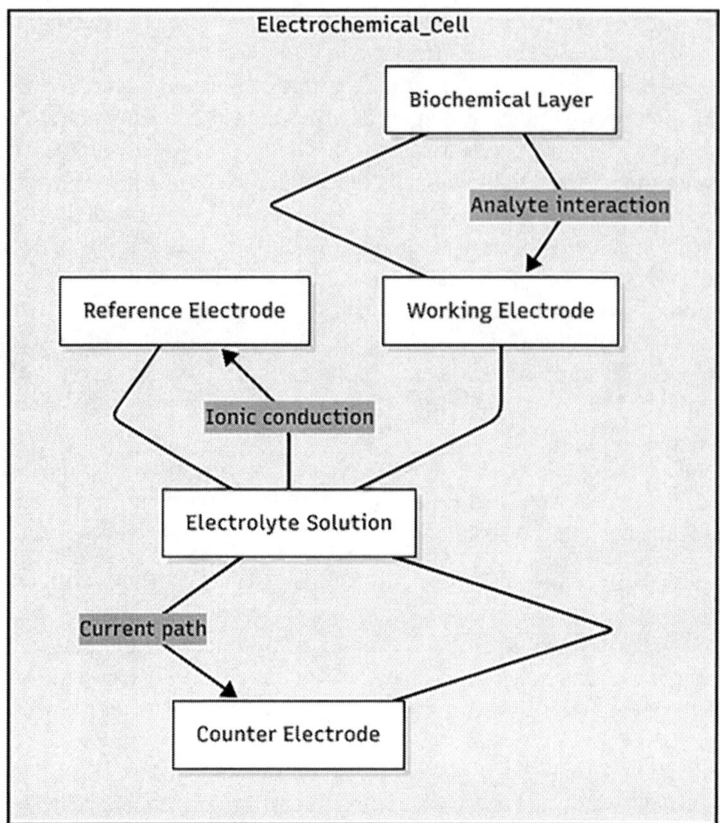

Fig. 2.4 Three-electrode electrochemical cell schematic

Table 2.2 Common electrode materials and characteristics

Electrode type	Material	Advantages	Limitations	Typical application
Working	Glassy carbon	Wide potential window	Brittle	Enzyme sensors
Working	Gold	Good conductivity, easy functionalization	Expensive	DNA biosensors
Reference	Ag/AgCl	Stable potential	Sensitive to Cl^- depletion	General use
Counter	Pt wire	Chemically inert	Cost	Universal counter

measures the resulting current. Both instruments are capable of performing a range of electrochemical measurement techniques, including cyclic voltammetry, linear sweep voltammetry, chronoamperometry, and electrochemical impedance spectroscopy (EIS). Together, they allow researchers to obtain a precise understanding of

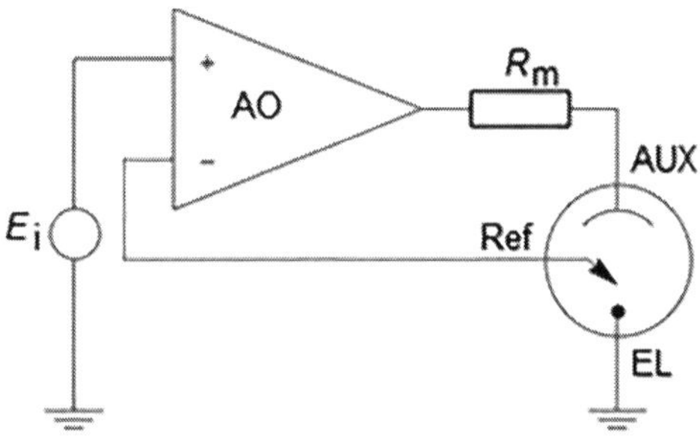

Fig. 2.5 Potentiostat (https://commons.wikimedia.org/wiki/File:Potentiostat_ro_1.png)

reaction kinetics, diffusion processes, and charge-transfer mechanisms occurring at the electrode interface (Fig. 2.5).

EIS is one of the most powerful analytical methods integrated into biosensor systems. EIS evaluates the impedance of an electrochemical system across a wide frequency range, providing insight into the dynamic behavior of the electrode–electrolyte interface. This method helps characterize reaction kinetics, mass transport phenomena, and the electrolyte's intrinsic resistance. Because it can distinguish between capacitive and resistive elements in the system, EIS is often employed to optimize biosensor performance, improve signal stability, and evaluate coating or membrane properties.

Advanced potentiostat and galvanostat systems are equipped with source/load boosters that enable them to handle high-current ranges, extending their utility to applications such as hydrogen fuel cells, electrolyzers, solid-oxide cells, and high-power lithium or redox-flow batteries [14]. These instruments can operate over a range of voltages and currents, making them suitable for both fundamental electrochemical research and applied testing environments.

Modern electrochemical software packages integrate numerous capabilities, including:

- Impedance spectroscopy: Measurement frequencies typically range from 1 mHz to 100 kHz, enabling precise modeling of complex electrochemical systems.
- Current control: Adjustable ranges that allow for micro- to macroampere current regulation to accommodate various biosensor designs.
- Cyclic voltammetry and chronoamperometry: Standard electrochemical techniques used for studying redox processes, electrode stability, and analyte diffusion.
- Automation and remote control: External operation via TCP/IP interfaces and compatibility with data acquisition platforms such as LabView, enabling automated experimental control and real-time data transfer.

These integrated software systems do not merely serve as analytical tools—they represent the central intelligence of the electrochemical biosensor setup. They control potential and current, continuously record data, apply mathematical models for data interpretation, and provide graphical visualization of results.

In practical applications, the combination of robust hardware and intelligent software creates a closed-loop system capable of performing highly precise electrochemical analyses with minimal user intervention. The automation and digitalization of data acquisition and processing have enabled more consistent results and facilitated the deployment of electrochemical biosensors across diverse fields, from medical diagnostics and pharmaceutical testing to environmental and industrial monitoring (Table 2.3).

Modern developments in electrochemical software continue to expand the range of techniques available for biosensor characterization. These include enhanced data-fitting algorithms for impedance spectra, real-time correction for environmental fluctuations, and integration with AImodels for predictive diagnostics. As a result, the software component of biosensing systems has become as essential as the physical transducer, ensuring reliability, reproducibility, and precision in every measurement.

Basic Electrochemical Principles

Electrochemical biosensing operates on the principles of redox reactions and the electrical phenomena that accompany electron transfer and ion movement. These interactions generate measurable signals that underpin biosensor functionality. Understanding how biosensors detect and quantify analytes requires familiarity with three fundamental electrochemical concepts: the Nernst equation, redox reactions, and current–voltage relationships.

The **Nernst equation** describes how the potential of an electrochemical cell depends on the concentrations of the reacting species in a redox reaction [15]. It allows prediction of electrode potentials under non-standard conditions, making it a cornerstone in interpreting biosensor responses. The equation is expressed as:

$$E = E^\circ - \frac{RT}{nF} \ln(Q) \tag{2.1}$$

Here, E represents the electrode potential, E° is the standard electrode potential, R is the gas constant, T is the absolute temperature, n is the number of electrons transferred, F is Faraday's constant, and Q is the reaction quotient reflecting the ratio of product to reactant concentrations. This relationship directly links analyte concentration to measurable electrical potential. In biosensing applications, the Nernst equation is used to calibrate sensors and interpret variations in voltage output as a function of target concentration.

Redox (reduction–oxidation) reactions serve as the chemical basis for electrochemical biosensors. These reactions involve electron exchange between two chemical species, one undergoing oxidation (electron loss) and the other reduction (electron gain). Within biosensors, this process often occurs following a biological recognition event, such as the catalytic reaction between an enzyme and its

Table 2.3 Main electrochemical techniques and their analytical purpose

Technique	Controlled parameter	Measured parameter	Application
Cyclic voltammetry	Potential sweep	Current	Redox mechanisms
Chronoamperometry	Step potential	Current vs time	Kinetic studies
EIS	AC frequency	Impedance	Surface characterization

substrate. As electrons are transferred to or from the electrode, the sensor records a change in current or potential that reflects the amount of analyte present. For instance, glucose biosensors rely on the oxidation of glucose by glucose oxidase, which produces electrons that are detected electrochemically.

The relationship between current and applied voltage governs the overall behavior of electrochemical biosensors. During redox reactions at the electrode surface, the current generated is influenced by the applied potential, reactant concentration, and the rate of mass transport by diffusion or convection [16]. Techniques such as cyclic voltammetry are often used to characterize this behavior. In cyclic voltammetry, a voltage sweep produces characteristic peaks that correspond to oxidation and reduction processes, allowing researchers to identify reaction kinetics and determine sensor sensitivity. Instruments such as potentiostats are used to precisely control the voltage and measure the resulting current, converting these electrochemical responses into quantifiable signals that form the basis of biosensor readings.

2.1.3 Types of Devices

Biosensors can be categorized based on the mechanism that provides biological specificity, the type of physical or chemical transduction involved, or a combination of both. From this perspective, the most common types of biosensors include amperometric, potentiometric, conductometric, and FET-based devices. Each of these systems operates using distinct principles for signal generation and detection, but all share the fundamental goal of converting a biological event into a measurable electrical signal.

Voltammetric and amperometric biosensors are among the most extensively used electrochemical devices for analytical detection due to their high sensitivity and rapid response. Their functionality relies on measuring the electrical current resulting from oxidation or reduction reactions occurring at the electrode surface. These reactions are catalyzed by biological elements such as enzymes that specifically recognize the target analyte.

In **voltammetric biosensors**, the applied potential varies over time, typically in a linear or cyclic manner, while in amperometric biosensors, the potential remains constant. Both systems measure the current produced as the analyte undergoes electrochemical transformation. The resulting current is directly proportional to the analyte concentration, providing quantitative information. Voltammetric techniques include cyclic voltammetry, linear sweep voltammetry, square wave voltammetry, and differential pulse voltammetry, each suited to different analytical purposes depending on sensitivity requirements and kinetic parameters. The high sensitivity of these biosensors arises from their ability to detect minute changes in electron flow caused by biochemical reactions. As a result, voltammetric and amperometric biosensors are widely used for clinical diagnostics, environmental monitoring, and food analysis. Their design flexibility and compatibility with miniaturized electrode systems make them particularly suitable for point-of-care applications.

Potentiometric biosensors operate using electrochemical cells that include at least two electrodes, often **ion-selective electrodes (ISEs).** These devices measure the potential difference generated by ionic activity in the vicinity of the sensing electrode, typically while drawing negligible current. Biological components such as enzymes are incorporated to catalyze reactions that either produce or consume ions near the electrode surface [17]. The resulting changes in ion concentration alter the potential, which is measured as the analytical signal. These sensors offer several advantages, including small size, fast response time, ease of use, and low manufacturing costs. They are relatively resistant to interference from sample color or turbidity and can function accurately across a range of sample volumes. Because of these attributes, potentiometric biosensors are promising candidates for point-of-care diagnostic applications. In recent research, novel potentiometric biosensors have been developed using extended-gate FET configurations, allowing dual-chip architectures for enhanced signal stability and miniaturization. Such designs have demonstrated successful application in rapid serological testing for viral infections and other biomedical assays.

Fluorescence-based biosensors have become increasingly prominent for detecting infectious diseases and biochemical targets due to their exceptional sensitivity, low cost, and rapid signal generation. These systems rely on fluorophores—fluorescent dyes or nanomaterials, that emit light upon excitation at a specific wavelength. The emitted fluorescence intensity correlates with the concentration of the target analyte. A common mechanism in fluorescence biosensing is **fluorescence resonance energy transfer (FRET),** in which energy is transferred from a donor fluorophore to an acceptor molecule in a distance-dependent manner. The occurrence and efficiency of this transfer serve as the basis for quantitative measurements. Advances in nanotechnology have further expanded the field by introducing fluorescent nanoparticles, quantum dots, and other materials capable of producing or modulating fluorescence signals with improved stability and brightness [18].

Fluorescence biosensors can be categorized according to how the signal changes upon target binding:

- In direct-labeling biosensors, the fluorescent tag is attached to a specific ligand that binds the target molecule, producing a signal proportional to the analyte concentration.
- In "signal-on" systems, fluorescence increases upon analyte binding.
- In "signal-off" systems, fluorescence intensity decreases when the analyte is present.

These approaches enable a range of detection strategies for rapid, precise, and sensitive quantification of biological markers, making fluorescence biosensors highly adaptable for clinical and environmental applications.

Magnetic biosensors use magnetic materials and phenomena to detect biological targets. Their operation is based on monitoring magnetic-field changes induced by magnetic particles or materials bound to the analyte. Compared with optical or electrochemical sensors, magnetic biosensors offer distinct advantages such as low background noise, since biological samples generally lack magnetic properties, and reduced sample preparation time, as magnetic fields can be used for rapid separation and concentration of analytes. These sensors demonstrate high specificity, sensitivity, and signal-to-noise ratios, making them ideal for point-of-care detection where speed and reliability are essential. Over the past few decades, several magnetic biosensor technologies have been developed, including giant magnetoresistance (GMR) biosensors, magnetic tunneling junctions, magnetic particle spectroscopy (MPS) systems, and nuclear magnetic resonance (NMR)-based sensors.

Among these, GMR and MPS biosensors have attracted significant attention for their ability to detect infectious agents and biomolecular targets at extremely low concentrations. The GMR effect, discovered in the 1980s, occurs in multilayer structures composed of alternating ferromagnetic and nonmagnetic materials [19]. Later findings demonstrated that this effect could also occur in homogeneous media such as granular films, broadening its applicability in biomedical sensing.

One of the main challenges associated with magnetic biosensing was the need for multiple washing steps during assay preparation, which increased assay time. Recent advances have addressed this issue by developing wash-free magnetic assays integrated into portable diagnostic platforms. These innovations have greatly simplified the testing process, reduced sample handling, and improved detection speed and accuracy—making magnetic biosensors an increasingly practical solution for real-world diagnostic use (Table 2.4).

2.1.4 Clinical Applications

A biosensor is broadly defined as a device that incorporates a biological recognition component, such as an enzyme, antibody, nucleic acid, microorganism, or tissue fragment, physically attached or confined to a transducer. This biological element provides the primary source of selectivity, enabling the biosensor to detect specific analytes through biochemical interactions. The accuracy, specificity, and sensitivity of a biosensor depend largely on the biological material and the method used to immobilize it onto the transducer surface. Several immobilization techniques have been developed to stabilize these biological components, including covalent

Table 2.4 Performance summary of major biosensor types

Sensor type	Transduction mode	Measured signal	Detection limit	Typical response time	Applications
Amperometric	Current	μA	10^{-6} M	1–10 s	Glucose
Potentiometric	Voltage	mV	10^{-4} M	<5 s	Urea
Impedimetric	Impedance	Ω	10^{-9} M	<60 s	Pathogen
FET	Conductance	nS	10^{-12} M	Real time	DNA probe

bonding, physical adsorption, cross-linking, encapsulation, and entrapment within polymer matrices [15, 20].

Biosensors function by converting biochemical reactions into quantifiable signals. Most biosensors employ electrochemical transducers, amperometric, potentiometric, or conductometric, which measure current, voltage, or conductivity changes resulting from the interaction between the analyte and the immobilized biological molecule. The core principle of these devices is that chemical reactions between the target analyte and the immobilized biomolecule result in the generation or consumption of ions or electrons, thereby producing measurable changes in electrical properties, such as current, potential, or impedance. Other biosensors utilize optical transducers, which detect variations in light intensity, fluorescence, or diffraction patterns resulting from analyte binding. Thermometric biosensors monitor the heat released or absorbed during biochemical reactions using temperature-sensitive elements. Mechanical biosensors, such as piezoelectric or microcantilever-based devices, measure physical changes, such as variations in mass, density, or viscosity, when biomolecules adsorb onto the sensor surface [21]. Among all these classes, electrochemical biosensors remain the most widely used due to their simplicity, low cost, high sensitivity, and suitability for miniaturization. Well-designed biosensors offer significant advantages in clinical and analytical contexts: high selectivity, rapid response time, low sample volume requirements, and ease of operation. They have become essential tools in medical diagnostics, environmental monitoring, and biotechnology. However, several challenges still hinder their large-scale commercial deployment. These include the instability of biological components, interference from non-target substances, limited reproducibility, and the need to simplify the device design for routine use by non-specialists.

Glucose measurement represents one of the most common applications of biosensor technology and remains the foundation for many modern point-of-care diagnostic systems. Monitoring glucose levels is crucial for the management of diabetes and other metabolic disorders. Normal physiological glucose concentrations typically range around 110 ± 25 mg/dL, while diabetic patients may experience values exceeding 360 mg/dL.

The **glucose biosensor** was the first biosensor ever developed. The concept originated in the early 1960s when the enzyme glucose oxidase (GOx) was immobilized on an oxygen electrode through a dialysis membrane. This setup enabled glucose detection by measuring oxygen consumption and hydrogen peroxide production during enzymatic oxidation. The reaction involves the conversion of β-D-glucose to gluconic acid, coupled with the reduction of oxygen to hydrogen peroxide. The resulting current, proportional to the analyte concentration, underlies amperometric glucose detection [22].

This type of biosensor revolutionized medical diagnostics, enabling diabetic patients to monitor their blood glucose levels independently. Modern glucose biosensors have evolved into compact, disposable devices with advanced features, including real-time wireless data transmission and continuous glucose monitoring via subcutaneous sensors.

Lactate biosensors are vital tools in clinical and physiological studies, as blood lactate levels are indicators of metabolic status and tissue oxygenation. Elevated lactate concentrations are associated with respiratory insufficiency, circulatory shock, cardiac failure, and metabolic disorders. **Amperometric biosensors for lactate detection** commonly employ lactate oxidase (LOX) or lactate dehydrogenase (LDH) immobilized on electrode surfaces. Advances in materials science have significantly improved their performance. For instance, incorporating multi-walled carbon nanotubes (MWCNTs) into sol–gel films enhances electron transfer between the enzyme and the electrode, thereby improving sensitivity and broadening the detection range. Biosensors with such modifications have demonstrated linear detection ranges of 0.2–2.0 mM and have been successfully applied to measure lactate levels in real human blood samples.

Cholesterol monitoring is of major clinical importance because elevated cholesterol levels are linked to cardiovascular diseases such as atherosclerosis, hypertension, coronary artery disease, and stroke. Maintaining cholesterol concentrations below approximately 5 mM significantly reduces the risk of these conditions. Most **cholesterol biosensors** use cholesterol oxidase (ChOX) as the biorecognition element, catalyzing the oxidation of cholesterol to cholest-4-en-3-one and hydrogen peroxide [23]. The generated hydrogen peroxide can be electrochemically detected, producing a current that correlates with cholesterol concentration. Such biosensors provide a fast, reliable, and cost-effective method for assessing lipid profiles and guiding therapeutic interventions.

Urea biosensors are used to monitor renal function and diagnose kidney-related diseases, such as acute renal failure and chronic kidney disease. The most common clinical tests, such as blood urea nitrogen (BUN) and urine urea nitrogen (UUN), measure urea levels in body fluids to assess kidney function. These biosensors typically rely on urease, an enzyme that catalyzes the hydrolysis of urea into ammonia and bicarbonate ions. The resulting changes in pH or ionic concentration can be measured electrochemically or potentiometrically. Although abnormal urea levels are not always indicative of renal dysfunction, they can also result from dehydration or excessive protein intake, biosensors for urea detection provide rapid, precise results that are valuable for both clinical diagnostics and biomedical research.

Nucleic acid biosensors have become essential tools in genetic diagnostics, forensic science, and molecular biology. These devices detect specific DNA or RNA sequences through hybridization reactions between a complementary nucleic acid probe immobilized on the sensor surface and the target sequence present in the sample. **Electrochemical DNA biosensors** can detect mutations, genetic disorders, and infectious agents by measuring changes in current, voltage, or impedance during hybridization events. They can also be used to monitor gene expression or evaluate the presence of pathogens in various environmental and clinical samples. The sensitivity and selectivity of DNA biosensors depend on the stability of the immobilized probe and the hybridization efficiency [24]. Continuous innovations in nanomaterials and signal amplification techniques, such as the use of redox-active intercalators, have further enhanced their detection capabilities, enabling the identification of genetic markers at extremely low concentrations (Table 2.5).

Table 2.5 Representative clinical biosensors and analytical parameters

Target analyte	Biological element	Transduction method	Linear range (mM)	LOD (mM)	Sample type
Glucose	Glucose oxidase	Amperometric	0.1–20	0.01	Blood
Lactate	Lactate oxidase	Amperometric	0.2–2	0.05	Serum
Cholesterol	Cholesterol oxidase	Amperometric	0.5–10	0.1	Plasma
Urea	Urease	Potentiometric	1–20	0.5	Urine

2.1.5 Regulatory Considerations

The development and commercialization of electrochemical biosensors require strict adherence to regulatory frameworks designed to ensure product safety, reliability, and performance. These regulations govern biosensors as either in vitro diagnostic (IVD) devices or medical devices, depending on their intended use, target population, and operating environment. Compliance with these standards is essential not only for market approval but also for ensuring consistent analytical accuracy and patient safety. The regulation of optical biosensors is primarily overseen by agencies such as the U.S. Food and Drug Administration (FDA), the European Medicines Agency (EMA), and comparable bodies, including Health Canada, the Pharmaceuticals and Medical Devices Agency (PMDA) in Japan, and the notified bodies within the European Union. These organizations classify medical devices based on risk and intended use, dictating the level of testing and documentation required before market approval. High-risk biosensors, such as those used to guide cancer treatment or detect life-threatening infections, undergo far more stringent validation procedures than lower-risk, over-the-counter diagnostic tools.

In the United States, biosensors are regulated by the FDA through the Center for Devices and Radiological Health (CDRH). Devices are classified according to their risk level, Class I, II, or III, with Class I representing low-risk general-use devices and Class III reserved for those that pose higher risk or involve life-supporting functions. Most electrochemical biosensors, particularly those used for point-of-care diagnostics such as glucose monitoring, typically fall under Class II. This category requires a premarket notification or 510(k) submission to demonstrate substantial equivalence to an already approved device [25].

In the European Union, biosensors are regulated under the In Vitro Diagnostic Regulation (IVDR) 2017/746, which came into effect in May 2022. The IVDR introduced a more rigorous classification system, with classes ranging from Class A to Class D, reflecting increasing risk levels. To be marketed within the EU, biosensors must obtain CE marking, which certifies conformity with applicable safety and performance standards. The conformity assessment process may involve clinical evaluations, technical documentation, and audits conducted by notified bodies. Depending on the device's complexity, the process may take several months to 2 years. Manufacturers must prepare detailed regulatory documentation, typically including an EU Declaration of Conformity, technical files, and, where necessary, an EC certificate issued by a notified body. These documents must remain valid throughout the product's lifecycle and be updated whenever significant modifications occur.

To achieve regulatory approval, biosensor manufacturers must demonstrate several key performance characteristics:

- Accuracy and Precision: The biosensor must produce results consistent with reference methods across repeated measurements.
- Linearity and Sensitivity: It should maintain linear responses across the expected range of analyte concentrations.
- Limit of Detection (LOD) and Limit of Quantification (LOQ): The smallest detectable and quantifiable concentrations of the analyte must be established under standardized testing conditions.
- Stability and Reproducibility: The biosensor must maintain performance over its intended shelf life and under defined storage conditions.

Biosensors that come into contact with biological fluids, such as blood, saliva, or sweat, must also comply with relevant ISO standards, particularly ISO 13485 for quality management systems and ISO 14971 for risk management in medical devices. These standards ensure that the design, manufacturing, and post-market surveillance processes follow internationally recognized best practices. Additionally, electrical safety and electromagnetic compatibility must be verified in accordance with IEC 60601-1 and IEC 60601-2, which define the safety requirements for electrical medical equipment. These standards ensure that biosensors do not pose electrical hazards and that their performance remains unaffected by electromagnetic interference (Fig. 2.6).

As biosensors increasingly incorporate digital technologies, software integration, and wireless connectivity, data security and cybersecurity have become critical aspects of regulatory compliance. Devices that process or transmit sensitive patient data must adhere to data integrity principles and follow the FDA's cybersecurity guidance for medical devices. This includes implementing secure communication protocols, encryption, and software update mechanisms to protect against unauthorized access or data manipulation.

Certain biosensors may be marketed as wellness devices rather than medical devices if they are intended for general health monitoring without diagnostic or therapeutic claims. However, once a biosensor claims to diagnose, prevent, or treat disease, it falls within the scope of medical device regulations and must undergo the appropriate conformity and approval procedures.

2.1.6 Future Perspectives

Over the past six decades, biosensors have evolved from conceptual devices into indispensable analytical tools for detecting a wide range of analytes across food, clinical, and environmental fields. The first generation of enzyme-based

Fig. 2.6 Regulatory approval pathway flowchart

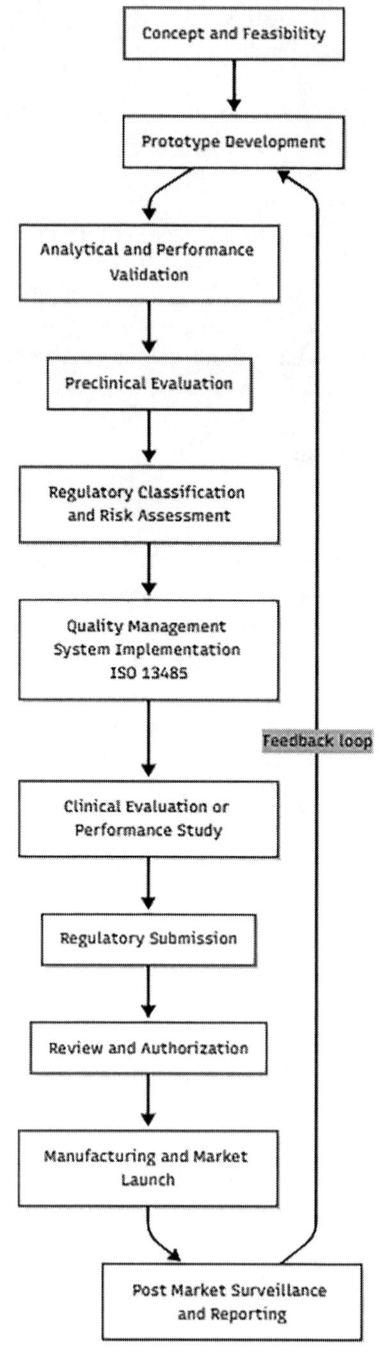
Concept and Feasibility
Prototype Development
Analytical and Performance Validation
Preclinical Evaluation
Regulatory Classification and Risk Assessment
Quality Management System Implementation ISO 13485
Feedback loop
Clinical Evaluation or Performance Study
Regulatory Submission
Review and Authorization
Manufacturing and Market Launch
Post Market Surveillance and Reporting

electrochemical biosensors, introduced in the early 1960s, established the foundation for modern biosensing technologies. Since then, the field has expanded to include biosensors that use antibodies, nucleic acids, cells, and synthetic recognition elements, driving ongoing innovation and diversification.

The growing number of scientific publications and technological developments reflects the increasing importance of biosensors in modern research and diagnostics. Today, the term biosensor encompasses a vast array of devices that differ in biological components, transduction mechanisms, and applications [26]. These include systems that employ catalytic biomolecules, such as enzymes and DNAzymes; abiotic materials with biocatalytic properties; aptamer-based sensors; and hybrid devices integrating both biological and synthetic recognition elements. The principles of transduction now extend beyond electrochemical mechanisms to include optical, magnetic, thermal, and piezoelectric systems, each tailored to specific analytical contexts.

Contemporary research also explores integrating biosensors into wearable and implantable platforms. These next-generation systems enable continuous, minimally invasive health monitoring by detecting biomarkers directly from body fluids, such as sweat, tears, saliva, or interstitial fluid. For example, continuous glucose monitoring devices represent a major success in wearable technology, allowing diabetic patients to track glucose levels in real time without frequent blood sampling. Such innovations are reshaping personalized medicine by facilitating early diagnosis, remote patient monitoring, and data-driven healthcare.

Wearable biosensors are increasingly combined with microfluidic systems that guide and process small volumes of biological fluids directly on the sensor's surface. This integration allows rapid transport, separation, and analysis of analytes without external laboratory equipment. By combining microfluidics with advanced materials and miniaturized electronics, researchers are creating compact and multifunctional biosensing platforms capable of wireless data transmission and cloud-based analysis.

Beyond clinical diagnostics, biosensors are finding applications in forensic science, biometric security, and environmental surveillance. In forensic analysis, biosensors can detect metabolites or biomarkers from trace biological samples, providing a faster alternative to traditional DNA-based identification methods. These technologies can provide valuable information about an individual's physiological state or the origin of a biological sample while avoiding the lengthy processes associated with DNA profiling (Fig. 2.7).

Parallel advancements in materials science have also opened new opportunities for photoelectrochemical biosensors, which couple biological recognition elements with semiconductor materials that generate electrical signals under light illumination. By combining enzymes such as acetylcholinesterase or glucose oxidase with semiconductor nanoparticles—like titanium dioxide or quantum dots—researchers have enhanced the sensitivity and signal stability of these hybrid systems [27]. Future developments in this area are expected to explore new semiconductor–biomolecule combinations and wavelength-tuning strategies to create multi-analyte

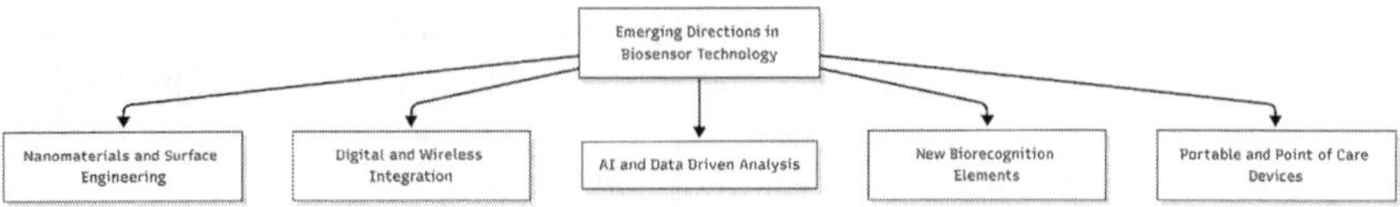

Fig. 2.7 Emerging biosensor technologies

photoelectrochemical sensors capable of simultaneous detection of several biomarkers.

Another major direction involves FET-based biosensors, particularly those built upon electrolyte–insulator–semiconductor (EIS) structures. These systems provide direct electronic readouts and represent a bridge between chemical sensing and semiconductor technology. They are being developed as part of a new generation of lab-on-a-chip devices, offering label-free detection and high integration potential for diagnostic applications. Advances in two-dimensional materials such as graphene, transition metal dichalcogenides (TMDCs), hexagonal boron nitride (h-BN), and black phosphorus have further improved FET biosensor performance by increasing surface area, electron mobility, and biocompatibility. These materials are enabling highly responsive, miniaturized biosensors that can detect ultralow analyte concentrations.

The future of biosensing lies in multifunctional, intelligent systems that combine multiple detection principles within a single device. Hybrid sensors that integrate electrochemical and optical transduction mechanisms, supported by AIand data analytics, are being designed to interpret complex biological information in real time. Such systems will be able to analyze multiple biomarkers simultaneously, identify disease patterns, and adapt to environmental or physiological changes.

Further progress will also depend on improving biocompatibility, signal stability, and long-term operational lifespan, particularly for implantable biosensors. Research efforts are increasingly focusing on surface modification techniques, antifouling coatings, and self-healing materials that preserve sensor performance in biological environments.

2.2 Optical Biosensors

In today's analytical and biotechnological landscape, optical biosensors have emerged as pivotal tools for detecting, monitoring, and analyzing a wide variety of biological and chemical substances. The growing demand for rapid, accurate, and sensitive diagnostic technologies across medicine, environmental monitoring, food safety, and homeland security has solidified their importance. These devices stand out for combining remarkable sensitivity and selectivity with the ability to perform real-time, often label-free detection.

At their foundation, optical biosensors consist of a biological recognition element, commonly antibodies, enzymes, nucleic acids, or aptamers, coupled with an optical transducer. The biological component ensures selectivity through specific interactions with the target analyte, while the optical transducer detects and translates these interactions into measurable signals. Such signals typically manifest as changes in light properties, including intensity, wavelength, polarization, or refractive index [28]. One of the defining advantages of optical biosensors is their capacity for non-invasive, real-time monitoring, a quality that makes them especially valuable in clinical diagnostics and environmental testing (Fig. 2.8).

The functional principle of these devices lies in how light interacts with the complex formed between the analyte and the bioreceptor. Several optical detection methods have been developed, each suited to particular applications. SPR enables real-time, label-free detection of molecular interactions and is a mainstay in pharmacological and biochemical research. Fluorescence-based biosensors, particularly those employing Förster resonance energy transfer, are frequently used in cell imaging and tracking dynamic molecular events. Other techniques such as interferometry, Raman spectroscopy, and photonic crystal sensing have expanded the scope and versatility of optical biosensing platforms.

Recent advances in nanotechnology, microfluidics, and material science have greatly enhanced the sensitivity and portability of these sensors. Incorporating nanostructures, such as gold nanoparticles, quantum dots, and graphene derivatives, has improved signal amplification, lowered detection limits, and shortened response times. The integration of optical biosensors into portable and wearable formats is also transforming diagnostics, enabling personalized and point-of-care testing even in settings with limited infrastructure.

Optical biosensors thus represent a field that unites biology, chemistry, physics, and engineering. Their capabilities are redefining the way biological systems are studied and monitored, offering solutions that are fast, selective, and minimally invasive. As ongoing research continues to push boundaries in sensitivity, specificity, and ease of use, these devices are set to play an even greater role in the future of scientific and technological innovation.

2.2.1 History

The origins of biosensors, and, by extension, optical biosensors, can be traced back to the development of analytical methods that combine biological recognition with physical transduction. The concept of a biosensor emerged in the 1960s, when scientists began integrating enzymes, antibodies, and other biological molecules into detection systems to achieve selective and sensitive analysis [29]. One of the earliest breakthroughs was the enzyme-based glucose electrode developed by Leland C. Clark Jr. and Champ Lyons in 1962, which set the foundation for modern biosensor technology. Although initially electrochemical, this innovation opened the path for optical transduction mechanisms that would later define the next generation of biosensing devices.

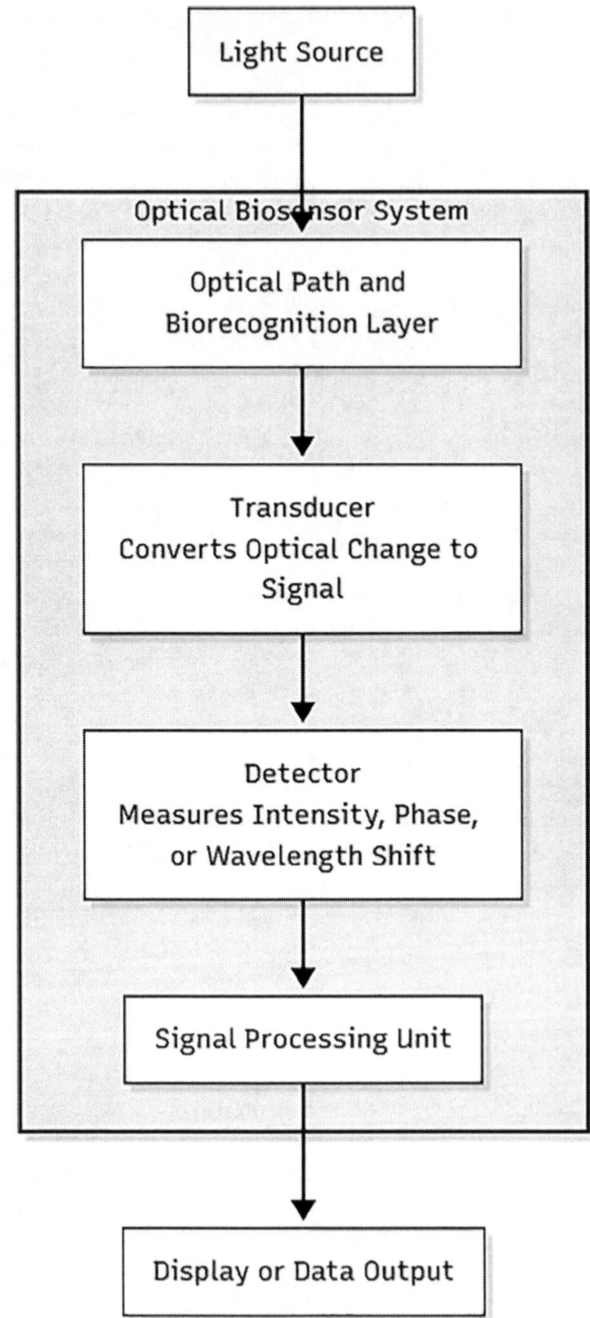

Fig. 2.8 General architecture of an optical biosensor

Optical biosensors gained attention in the 1970s, fueled by advances in laser sources, fiber optics, and photodetectors that enabled more precise light-based measurements. These systems work by detecting the interaction between light and biological analytes, producing measurable changes in absorbance, fluorescence, luminescence, or refractive index. One of the earliest successful optical biosensors used fiber-optic fluorescence technology to monitor chemical and biological parameters such as pH and dissolved gases. These early developments demonstrated the feasibility of in vivo monitoring and paved the way for miniaturized, flexible sensors capable of operating in complex environments. As optical components such as laser diodes and photomultiplier tubes became more reliable and affordable during the 1980s, optical biosensors transitioned from experimental prototypes to practical analytical instruments used in biomedical and environmental applications.

A defining milestone in optical biosensing came with the introduction of surface plasmon resonance. This technique measures changes in the refractive index near a thin metallic surface, often gold, when light interacts with surface plasmons. When biomolecular binding occurs at the sensor interface, the refractive index changes, altering the resonance condition [30]. This enables label-free, real-time analysis of binding events, such as antigen–antibody reactions. By the early 1990s, commercial SPR-based instruments transformed molecular interaction analysis, particularly in drug discovery and immunology. These systems provided direct, kinetic information on molecular binding, becoming essential tools for understanding biomolecular mechanisms. SPR technology remains a cornerstone of optical biosensing today and continues to evolve toward smaller, more integrated, and more automated platforms.

Parallel to SPR advancements, fluorescence-based biosensors experienced rapid development. These systems use fluorescent labels or proteins that emit light upon excitation at specific wavelengths, enabling highly sensitive detection of biological interactions. The introduction of molecular probes such as green fluorescent protein and synthetic fluorophores in the 1990s enabled more sophisticated methods, including fluorescence resonance energy transfer and lifetime-based sensing. These tools allowed researchers to study live-cell dynamics, protein interactions, and enzyme activity with unparalleled precision. Fluorescence-based biosensing also found applications in genomics and proteomics, where DNA microarrays and fluorescent immunoassays became standard methods for gene expression and protein profiling. The ability to visualize and quantify molecular interactions in real time established fluorescence as one of the most versatile and widely adopted optical detection techniques.

The 2000s brought transformative changes as nanotechnology and photonics merged with biosensor design. Nanostructured materials, such as gold nanoparticles, quantum dots, and carbon nanomaterials, were introduced to enhance sensitivity and signal transduction. Gold nanoparticles, in particular, proved valuable for amplifying plasmonic and colorimetric signals, while quantum dots offered high brightness and tunable emission for multiplexed detection. Graphene and carbon nanotubes improved conductivity and biocompatibility, thereby enhancing sensor stability and performance.

The advent of photonic crystals, interferometric structures, and plasmonic waveguides further expanded biosensor functionality by enabling nanoscale control of light propagation. These technologies have since formed the backbone of high-sensitivity, label-free detection systems suitable for complex biological analyses [31]. In recent years, research has focused on creating portable, affordable, and user-friendly optical biosensors for point-of-care and field applications. The integration of microfluidics and optical detection into compact devices enables rapid testing with minimal sample volumes. Smartphones now serve as portable analyzers, using built-in cameras and light sources to measure fluorescence or colorimetric responses.

2.2.2   Technical Characteristics

Optical biosensors are complex analytical instruments designed to detect specific biological or chemical substances by capturing precise interactions between a biologically active component and an optical detection system. Their design integrates multiple functional layers, each contributing to the device's overall sensitivity, selectivity, and stability. At the center of this system is the biorecognition element, which provides molecular specificity and dictates the biosensor's selectivity. The performance of the entire biosensor depends on how efficiently this biological element recognizes and binds the target analyte, and how effectively the optical system converts that binding event into a measurable signal.

Biorecognition elements are typically immobilized on a solid substrate that forms part of the optical transducer. Immobilization must preserve biological activity and maintain stable binding to the surface while allowing sufficient interaction with the analyte. Several immobilization techniques are used, including physical adsorption, covalent attachment, cross-linking, and entrapment in polymeric or sol–gel matrices [32]. The choice of method affects not only the biosensor's sensitivity and durability but also its reusability. Different biological recognition elements are employed depending on the type of analyte and the intended application. Enzymes are among the most widely used components, serving as biocatalysts that produce optically detectable products. A classic example is glucose oxidase, which reacts with glucose to generate intermediates measurable through optical changes. This principle underlies many clinical glucose sensors. Antibodies represent another major class of biorecognition molecules, valued for their exceptional specificity and strong affinity for corresponding antigens. They are extensively used in immunosensors for medical diagnostics, environmental testing, and food analysis. Their versatility allows for the detection of viruses, toxins, and disease biomarkers with high confidence. Nucleic acid-based biosensors use single-stranded DNA or RNA probes that hybridize with complementary sequences, enabling precise detection of genetic material, mutations, or microbial DNA. When combined with optical techniques such as fluorescence or surface plasmon resonance, these sensors can monitor molecular hybridization in real time without the need for labels. Aptamers, synthetic oligonucleotides or peptides selected for specific molecular targets—have become an important alternative to antibodies. They can be tailored to bind small molecules, ions, or even entire cells, offering high specificity with improved chemical stability [33]. Because they are synthetically produced, aptamers reduce variability between batches and tolerate more extreme conditions, making them ideal for use in environmental or industrial biosensing. In certain cases, entire living cells or tissue fragments act as recognition elements. These cell-based biosensors are particularly valuable in toxicology and pharmacology, as they can detect toxins or drugs by measuring measurable biochemical or physiological changes. Although more complex to maintain, they more accurately mimic biological systems than isolated biomolecules, providing a realistic model of cellular responses.

Once a biological interaction occurs, whether enzymatic, immunological, nucleic acid hybridization, or cellular response, the optical transducer translates this event into an optical signal. The transducer operates on principles such as absorbance, fluorescence, luminescence, refractive index variation, or scattering. Each mechanism offers distinct advantages depending on the detection requirement. The precision and stability of the biological recognition process largely determine the biosensor's analytical performance. This integration of biological and optical components makes it suitable for applications ranging from medical diagnostics to environmental monitoring. As new recognition molecules and immobilization strategies emerge, the accuracy and sensitivity of optical biosensors continue to improve, broadening their relevance in both laboratory and field settings. The optical transducer serves as the link between biological recognition and the generation of a measurable signal. It converts the molecular interaction occurring on the biosensor surface into an optical response. Several modes of light interaction are employed for this purpose, including absorbance, fluorescence, chemiluminescence, surface plasmon resonance, interferometry, and Raman scattering [34]. Each approach has its own detection strengths depending on whether qualitative or quantitative information is required. The substrate on which the biorecognition element is immobilized is equally important. Common materials include glass, gold, silicon, and various polymers. The immobilization matrix must maintain the biological element's integrity while ensuring optimal light transmission or reflection. Advanced surface modifications and nanostructuring are often applied to enhance binding efficiency and optical performance.

Optical biosensors rely on various detection principles that translate biological binding events into measurable light-based changes. Each method harnesses a different physical property of light to detect biochemical interactions with high sensitivity and temporal precision. SPR is one of the most established and reliable methods in optical biosensing. Polarized light is directed onto a thin metallic film at a specific angle. When binding occurs on the metal surface, the refractive index changes, thereby shifting the resonance angle or wavelength. This shift can be directly measured, enabling real-time, label-free detection of biomolecular interactions. SPR is widely used to study binding kinetics, making it indispensable in drug discovery and molecular biology. Fluorescence-based detection relies on fluorophores that emit light upon excitation at a specific wavelength. Binding events can alter fluorescence intensity, emission wavelength, polarization, or lifetime. These variations are then quantified to determine analyte concentration. Advanced techniques such as Förster Resonance Energy Transfer and fluorescence polarization enable researchers to monitor molecular conformations, proximity, and dynamics within living cells [35]. Fluorescence detection offers extremely high sensitivity and enables multiplexed analysis of multiple analytes in a single sample.

Interferometric biosensors exploit light's wave nature to measure minute changes in optical path length. A light beam is split into two parts, one interacts with the sensing surface while the other serves as a reference. When the two beams recombine, the resulting interference pattern shifts in response to binding events on the sensor surface. Because of its ability to detect nanometer-scale changes, interferometry is well-suited for analyzing small molecules or low-concentration samples.

Raman spectroscopy, and its enhanced form, SERS provide another avenue for optical detection. When light interacts with molecules, most photons scatter elastically, but a small portion scatter inelastically, shifting energy as they do so. This inelastic scattering generates a spectral fingerprint unique to each molecule. When nanostructured metallic surfaces are used to amplify this signal, even trace levels of the analyte can be detected. Raman-based techniques are especially valuable for molecular identification and analysis in complex matrices.

Colorimetric detection offers a simpler, more accessible approach. It depends on visually observable color changes resulting from analyte binding, often via nanoparticle aggregation or enzymatic reactions. Although less sensitive than other optical methods, colorimetric biosensors are easy to interpret, inexpensive, and well-suited for rapid, point-of-care or field testing.

Together, these detection principles provide a comprehensive toolkit for designing biosensors that meet the requirements of different analytical contexts, whether ultra-sensitive laboratory assays or user-friendly portable diagnostics. The analytical performance of an optical biosensor is characterized by several key parameters that define its reliability, speed, and precision [36].

- Sensitivity describes the device's capacity to detect small changes in analyte concentration. It is influenced by both the efficiency of the biorecognition process and the amplification mechanisms used in the optical transducer. High-performance biosensors can detect analytes at concentrations as low as the pico- or nanomolar range.
- Specificity refers to the biosensor's ability to discriminate the target analyte from similar molecules. This parameter depends on the recognition element's binding affinity and selectivity. Minimizing cross-reactivity is essential, particularly when analyzing complex biological samples.
- Dynamic range represents the span between the lowest and highest detectable analyte concentrations. A broad dynamic range ensures the sensor remains effective across a wide range of sample concentrations without signal saturation or loss of resolution.
- Response time measures how quickly a biosensor reaches signal stability after analyte introduction. In applications requiring rapid decision-making, such as

clinical diagnostics or environmental monitoring, short response times are critical.

- Reproducibility and stability ensure that results remain consistent over repeated measurements and extended storage. Factors influencing stability include immobilization strategy, environmental conditions, and degradation of biological components.
- Regeneration and reusability contribute to cost efficiency. After detection, biosensors can often be regenerated by removing the bound analyte using controlled pH or ionic changes, allowing repeated use without loss of sensitivity.

Modern optical biosensors integrate several instrumental components that manage light generation, guidance, detection, and data analysis. Light sources may include LEDs, lasers, or broadband lamps, depending on the detection principle. Waveguides and optical fibers direct light efficiently through the system, while filters and lenses control wavelength selection and focus. Detectors such as photodiodes, photomultiplier tubes, CCDs, or CMOS sensors convert light into measurable electrical signals.

Signal amplification mechanisms, ranging from enzyme-catalyzed reactions to plasmonic nanoparticle enhancement, boost detection limits. The addition of microfluidic systems further refines precision by controlling fluid flow and minimizing sample consumption. Data acquisition software processes raw optical signals through calibration, noise filtering, and kinetic modeling. Increasingly, AI and ML algorithms are being integrated to enhance interpretation accuracy, automate pattern recognition, and predict outcomes based on complex datasets.

Hardware

The performance of an optical biosensor depends not only on the precision of its biological and optical components but also on the sophistication of its hardware architecture. The hardware defines how effectively the sensor can control, detect, and process light to capture subtle biochemical interactions. Each component, from the light source to the detector, must be designed to work in harmony, ensuring accurate signal generation, transmission, and interpretation under various operational conditions.

At the heart of every optical biosensor lies the light source, the driving element that produces the illumination needed to generate optical signals. The type of light source is selected based on the detection principle and the specific analyte being measured. Light-emitting diodes (LEDs) are common in compact, portable biosensing systems because they offer narrow emission spectra, low energy consumption, and excellent stability. Their affordability and long lifespan make them ideal for continuous monitoring applications. In contrast, systems requiring high-intensity or monochromatic light, such as SPR or Raman spectroscopy, depend on laser diodes. Lasers deliver coherent, directional light with very narrow spectral widths, enabling precise excitation of target molecules and improving measurement accuracy [23, 37]. For applications that require a broad spectral range, such as absorbance or spectral analysis, xenon and halogen lamps are often used for their wide spectral coverage and stable output.

The pathway that light follows through the biosensor is equally crucial. The optical path is shaped and directed by mirrors, lenses, and filters that control focus, wavelength, and polarization. Beam splitters divide the light into reference and measurement beams for differential detection, while gratings or waveguides manipulate light propagation in integrated systems. In miniaturized or flexible sensors, optical fibers serve as both light conduits and sensing elements. These fibers transmit light efficiently over long distances and can be functionalized to interact directly with the analyte. Depending on the application, single-mode fibers are used for high-resolution sensing, whereas multimode fibers are preferred when greater light intensity or simpler alignment is required.

After interacting with the biorecognition layer, the light must be captured and converted into an electrical signal. This process is carried out by photodetectors, which detect changes in light intensity, wavelength, or phase. Photodiodes are among the most widely used detectors due to their compact design, low noise, and rapid response. For applications requiring higher sensitivity, avalanche photodiodes (APDs) and photomultiplier tubes (PMTs) are employed. PMTs can detect extremely weak light signals, down to the single-photon level, making them valuable for fluorescence- and chemiluminescence-based biosensors. However, their relatively large size and high voltage requirements limit their use in portable or wearable devices (Table 2.6).

For applications involving spatial or spectral imaging, such as mapping fluorescence intensity or measuring distributed binding events, charge-coupled device (CCD) and complementary metal-oxide-semiconductor (CMOS) cameras are used. These imaging detectors provide high spatial resolution and enable the visualization of optical signals across two-dimensional sensor surfaces. When coupled with spectrometers, they can also analyze the full wavelength profile of emitted or reflected light, providing richer datasets for quantitative interpretation.

The signals generated by detectors are typically weak and susceptible to noise, necessitating careful signal conditioning before analysis. Electronic circuits within the biosensor amplify, filter, and digitize these signals. Amplifiers strengthen low-intensity signals, while filters remove unwanted noise and interference. Analog-to-digital converters (ADCs) transform the continuous light-derived signal into digital data that can be processed by microcontrollers or embedded processors [17, 38].

Table 2.6 Common light sources and detectors in optical biosensors

Component	Example type	Wavelength range (nm)	Advantages	Common application
Light source	LED	400–700	Compact, low power	Fluorescence, absorbance
Laser diode	630–1550	High coherence	SPR, Raman	
Detector	Photodiode	400–1100	Fast response	Absorbance
CCD/CMOS camera	400–900	Imaging, high throughput	Fluorescence, interferometry	
Photomultiplier tube (PMT)	200–800	High sensitivity	Low-light detection	

These processors are programmed to manage timing, control light sources, perform real-time analysis, and maintain stable operation across varying environmental conditions. Recent advances in embedded systems have allowed optical biosensors to become more intelligent and autonomous. Microcontrollers such as Arduino, STM32, and Raspberry Pi are commonly integrated into biosensor systems, providing programmable control over light modulation, data processing, and communication. These controllers can execute automated calibration, detect errors, and manage temperature or power regulation. The growing incorporation of wireless communication technologies such as Bluetooth, Wi-Fi, and near-field communication (NFC) enables biosensors to transmit data directly to computers, smartphones, or cloud databases, supporting real-time monitoring and telemedicine applications.

Mechanical design and the physical housing also play important roles in maintaining biosensor performance. The enclosure must protect delicate optical and electronic components from environmental disturbances such as dust, humidity, or mechanical shock. Materials like aluminum, polymer composites, or coated glass are commonly used for casings, depending on whether the device is intended for laboratory, clinical, or field use. The housing often includes thermal management features to prevent temperature fluctuations from affecting measurement stability.

One of the most promising directions in biosensor hardware development is the creation of integrated lab-on-a-chip platforms. These systems combine optics, microfluidics, and electronics into a single compact device, allowing complex analyses with small sample volumes. Microfluidic channels deliver and mix liquids with precision, while optical sensors simultaneously detect multiple analytes. These miniaturized systems offer portability, automation, and reduced reagent consumption, making them ideal for point-of-care testing and field diagnostics. Power management is another important consideration. Depending on the intended use, optical biosensors may be powered by rechargeable lithium-ion batteries, USB connections, or solar energy. For wearable or implantable devices, energy efficiency is critical. Advances in low-power electronics and adaptive signal processing have extended battery life without compromising sensitivity or accuracy.

The hardware of modern optical biosensors is the result of multidisciplinary engineering that integrates optics, electronics, microfabrication, and materials science. Each component, from the choice of light source and detector to the data processor and physical casing, contributes to achieving reliable, precise, and high-throughput detection. As biosensor technology continues to evolve, hardware design will remain a central area of innovation, driving the transition from laboratory-based systems to fully integrated, portable, and intelligent diagnostic tools.

Software
While the hardware of an optical biosensor provides the physical framework necessary for signal generation and detection, it is the software that gives the system intelligence, coordination, and analytical capability. Software determines how the biosensor operates, manages data, and interacts with users. It converts raw optical information into meaningful analytical results and enables automation, precision control, and real-time decision-making.

At its core, the software serves as the bridge connecting biological recognition events to interpretable outcomes. It controls the hardware elements, such as light sources, detectors, actuators, and microfluidic components, ensuring synchronization between illumination, data capture, and signal processing. Embedded software, or firmware, written in languages such as C or C++ runs on microcontrollers or microprocessors and handles low-level operations governing timing, calibration, and communication between modules. This control ensures that light modulation, signal collection, and fluid handling occur seamlessly and reproducibly.

Once the optical signals are captured, software takes on the critical role of signal processing. The raw data obtained from detectors often contains noise, background interference, or baseline drift. Specialized algorithms are applied to clean and refine the data, enhancing signal-to-noise ratio and measurement reliability. Common techniques include digital filtering, baseline correction, normalization, and smoothing using mathematical models such as Savitzky–Golay filters or Fourier transforms [25]. These preprocessing steps enable the biosensor to deliver accurate, stable outputs even under fluctuating environmental or experimental conditions.

For imaging-based biosensors that use detectors such as CCD or CMOS cameras, the software also performs advanced image processing. This involves analyzing pixel intensity, identifying regions of interest, tracking temporal fluorescence changes, or detecting shifts in emission peaks. Open-source tools and libraries such as OpenCV, ImageJ, and scikit-image are often integrated for real-time feature extraction and quantification. By transforming visual data into numerical information, these algorithms allow for the measurement of binding kinetics, concentration gradients, and spatial molecular distributions.

Control software also manages the biosensor's physical systems, particularly in platforms incorporating microfluidics or temperature regulation. It governs fluid movement, ensures uniform sample delivery, and maintains optimal reaction conditions. Feedback loops and control algorithms dynamically adjust parameters to maintain stable performance. High-speed applications may rely on real-time operating systems (RTOS) or field-programmable gate arrays (FPGAs), which provide rapid response times and deterministic operation, critical for time-sensitive assays (Fig. 2.9).

Beyond data acquisition, the analytical power of biosensor software lies in its ability to extract meaningful biological insights. After preprocessing, algorithms identify patterns such as shifts in absorbance or fluorescence intensity, spectral peak changes, or kinetic constants derived from binding curves. In applications such as surface plasmon resonance, the software models molecular interactions using established biochemical equations, such as Langmuir or Michaelis–Menten kinetics, to determine association, dissociation, and equilibrium constants. Programs such as MATLAB, Origin, or custom Python scripts are frequently used to automate this curve fitting and quantify interaction strength.

ML and AI have become integral to modern biosensor software design. As optical biosensors generate increasingly large datasets, especially in multiplexed or continuous monitoring applications, AI-driven models are used to classify binding events, identify anomalies, and predict outcomes. Algorithms such as Principal

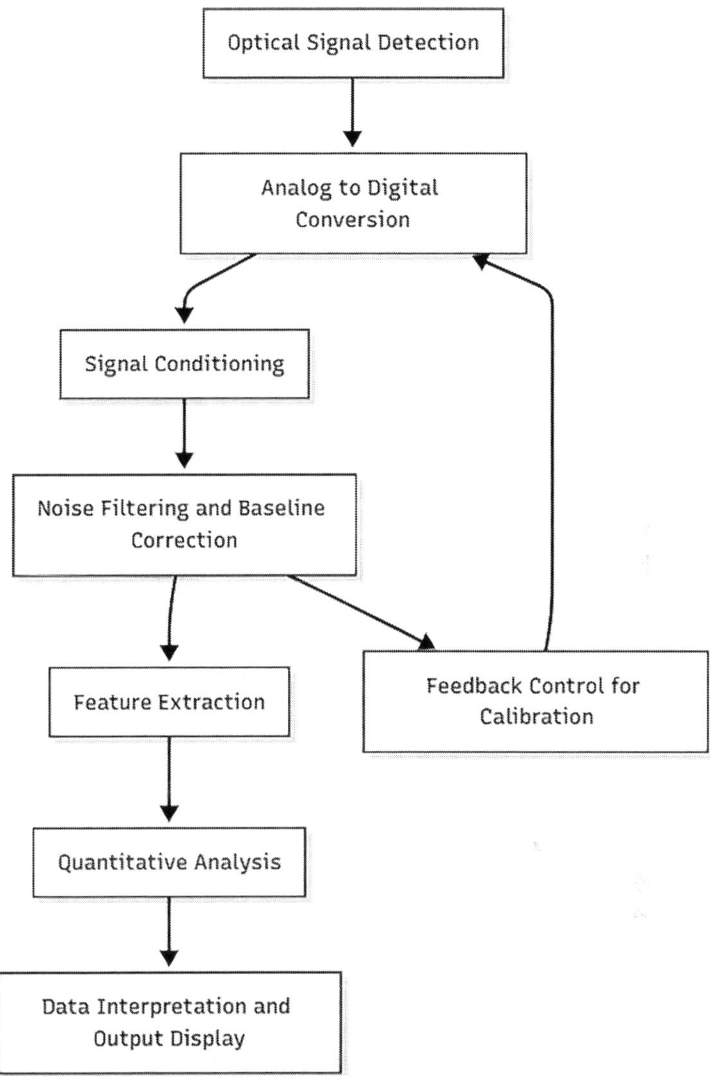

Fig. 2.9 Signal processing workflow in optical biosensors

Component Analysis (PCA) and Partial Least Squares (PLS) regression are applied for multivariate calibration, improving accuracy and robustness [9]. Deep learning frameworks like TensorFlow and PyTorch allow the biosensor to adapt to complex, non-linear data patterns, effectively transforming it into a self-optimizing analytical system capable of continuous improvement through data exposure.

User interaction is another essential aspect of biosensor software. Intuitive graphical user interfaces (GUIs) allow researchers or clinicians to operate the sensor, visualize results, and manage experiments without extensive training. GUIs provide real-time feedback through plots, heat maps, or numerical readouts, and often guide users through calibration or maintenance routines. Platforms like LabVIEW, MATLAB App Designer, and Python-based frameworks such as PyQt or Tkinter are commonly used to create these interfaces.

Many modern optical biosensors also include web-based or mobile applications that extend their usability beyond the laboratory. These interfaces enable remote control and data access through smartphones or computers. Built with technologies such as JavaScript, HTML5, and frameworks like React or Flask, these applications support cloud-based data storage and collaborative analysis. Through cloud platforms like ThingSpeak, Google Firebase, or Microsoft Azure, biosensors can transmit and process data in real time, allowing clinicians or researchers to monitor systems from anywhere in the world.

Calibration and diagnostic modules are built into the software to ensure long-term precision and reliability. Automated routines apply stored calibration curves, check for drift, and perform internal diagnostics to detect sensor degradation or contamination. If deviations are detected, the system alerts the user or performs self-correction. Data from these diagnostics can be stored in logs for regulatory reporting or quality assurance. Data management and security are also fundamental components of biosensor software. Depending on the application, information can be stored locally, in encrypted databases, or on secure cloud servers. Compliance with privacy regulations such as HIPAA or GDPR is essential, especially when biosensors handle medical data. Encryption protocols, user authentication, and data anonymization are implemented to protect sensitive information while maintaining traceability and data integrity.

In advanced healthcare and laboratory settings, biosensor software must also integrate seamlessly with other digital systems. This includes electronic health records (EHRs), laboratory information management systems (LIMS), and mobile health applications. Such integration requires adherence to standardized communication protocols like HL7 or FHIR, allowing biosensors to become part of interconnected healthcare ecosystems.

Emerging trends in biosensor software design are rapidly expanding the technology's capabilities. Edge computing enables localized data processing on devices, reducing latency and reliance on the internet. Blockchain technologies are being explored for secure traceability of health data and device performance history. Digital twin simulations, virtual representations of biosensors, allow developers to predict device behavior, optimize performance, and detect faults before they occur [10, 38]. Meanwhile, augmented reality interfaces are being developed to assist clinicians in interpreting sensor data during real-time patient monitoring (Table 2.7).

Ultimately, software transforms an optical biosensor from a collection of hardware components into an intelligent analytical system capable of autonomous operation and adaptive decision-making. As the integration of AI, connectivity, and real-time computation continues to advance, software will remain the defining factor in how effectively optical biosensors serve medicine, research, and industry.

Table 2.7 Software functions and associated tools

Function	Description	Example tools/Languages
Data acquisition	Controls light sources, sensors	C/C++, LabVIEW
Signal processing	Filtering, normalization, peak analysis	MATLAB, Python (NumPy, SciPy)
Image analysis	Region detection, intensity mapping	OpenCV, ImageJ
	Classification, regression	TensorFlow, PyTorch
GUI design	User interface and visualization	PyQt, Tkinter, App Designer
Cloud integration	Remote access, storage	Firebase, Azure, ThingSpeak

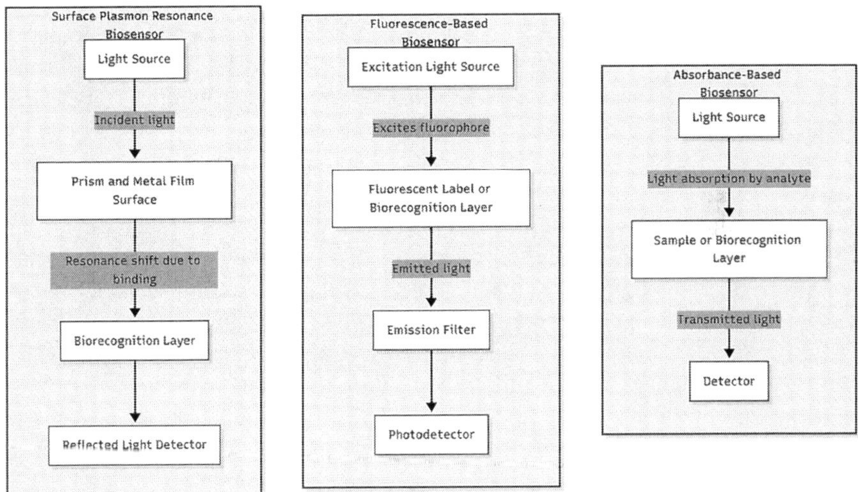

Fig. 2.10 Optical biosensors comparison

2.2.3 Types of Devices

Optical biosensors encompass several distinct categories of devices, each defined by its detection mechanism, optical configuration, and range of applications. Although these technologies differ in design and principle, they all share a common objective: translating biological recognition events into quantifiable optical signals. The diversity of optical biosensors allows them to meet the varied needs of biomedical research, clinical diagnostics, environmental testing, and industrial monitoring (Fig. 2.10).

SPR biosensors remain one of the most widely used and thoroughly studied types of optical biosensors. They operate based on the excitation of surface plasmons—coherent electron oscillations—on a thin metallic film, typically gold, when exposed to polarized light at a specific angle. When molecules bind to the sensor surface, the local refractive index changes, altering the resonance conditions. This shift is measured optically and corresponds directly to the amount of material bound to the surface. The primary advantage of SPR biosensors is their ability to provide real-time, label-free detection of biomolecular interactions. Unlike methods that require fluorescent or radioactive labeling, SPR can monitor the binding kinetics of proteins, antibodies, nucleic acids, or ligands directly as they occur. These systems are highly valued in pharmaceutical research for evaluating drug-receptor interactions, determining binding affinities, and characterizing molecular mechanisms. The development of commercial SPR instruments has made this technology a standard in academic and industrial laboratories alike, offering detailed kinetic profiles that help researchers design more effective therapeutics.

Fluorescence-based biosensors constitute another major category, using light-emitting molecules, or fluorophores, to detect specific analytes. When a fluorophore is excited by light of a particular wavelength, it emits light at a different wavelength. This emission changes in intensity, wavelength, or lifetime when the fluorophore interacts with a target molecule. Because of their exceptional sensitivity and versatility, fluorescence-based biosensors are used across many disciplines, including cellular biology, genetic analysis, and clinical diagnostics. They are particularly effective for detecting low-abundance analytes and for multiplexing, where several analytes are measured simultaneously in the same sample. In molecular biology, fluorescence biosensors are used to study real-time cellular events, such as enzyme activity, ion flux, and protein-protein interactions [23]. The incorporation of fluorescent proteins, synthetic dyes, or quantum dots allows for tunable emission spectra and compatibility with high-throughput imaging systems. Advanced devices in this category can track multiple biomarkers in a single assay, making fluorescence biosensing one of the most dynamic tools in analytical biotechnology.

Interferometric biosensors utilize the principle of light interference to detect molecular binding events. In these systems, a beam of light is divided into two paths—one interacts with the sensing surface, while the other serves as a reference. When the two beams recombine, their interference pattern changes with variations in the optical path length caused by analyte binding. Even small molecular interactions can induce detectable phase shifts or intensity modulations. This approach is highly sensitive and label-free, capable of detecting nanometer-scale changes in surface thickness or refractive index. Interferometric biosensors are often used to study drug-receptor binding, detect low-molecular-weight compounds, and analyze biomolecular interactions that are difficult to tag. The simplicity and precision of this method make it suitable for both research and industrial applications that require quantitative, real-time monitoring.

Optical fiber biosensors rely on the light-guiding properties of thin optical fibers to perform detection. These fibers can transmit light over long distances with minimal loss and are flexible enough to be incorporated into remote or in vivo sensing systems. The fiber surface is typically functionalized with a biorecognition layer, such as enzymes, antibodies, or aptamers, that specifically binds the analyte. When the analyte binds to the recognition element, it alters the optical properties of the transmitted or reflected light, producing measurable changes in intensity, phase, or wavelength. The inherent flexibility, small diameter, and resistance to electromagnetic interference make optical fiber biosensors ideal for use in environments where conventional optical setups would be impractical [16]. They are particularly useful in medical diagnostics, environmental monitoring, and industrial process control. In recent years, lab-on-fiber platforms have emerged, integrating microfluidics and photonic components directly onto the fiber surface to achieve real-time, high-throughput biosensing in extremely compact designs.

Photonic crystal biosensors utilize structured dielectric materials with periodic refractive index variations that control how light propagates within them. These photonic crystals reflect specific wavelengths of light, creating sharp resonance peaks that shift when the local refractive index changes due to biomolecular binding. This principle enables highly sensitive, label-free detection of analytes, making photonic crystal biosensors particularly valuable for biomedical diagnostics, food safety testing, and pharmaceutical screening. Their planar configuration facilitates integration into compact devices and microfluidic systems. The precision and tunability of photonic crystals also make them attractive for multiplexed detection platforms that can monitor multiple targets simultaneously.

Raman-based optical biosensors operate on the principle of inelastic scattering, in which photons interacting with molecules undergo energy shifts corresponding to specific vibrational modes. Each molecule produces a unique Raman spectrum, effectively serving as a molecular fingerprint. This feature enables Raman-based sensors not only to detect but also to identify substances with high specificity. When combined with nanostructured metallic surfaces, the Raman signal can be dramatically amplified, a phenomenon known as SERS. This enhancement allows the detection of molecules at extremely low concentrations, even down to single-molecule levels. Raman biosensors are widely applied in medical diagnostics, environmental analysis, and food safety. They are particularly useful for detecting cancer biomarkers, identifying pathogens, and assessing chemical contamination in complex biological or environmental samples. The distinguishing strength of Raman-based biosensors lies in their ability to provide structural information about the analyte without the need for labels or dyes. Their multiplexing capacity and robustness make them valuable in both clinical and research settings, where accurate molecular characterization is essential (Table 2.8).

2.2.4   Clinical Applications

Optical biosensors have become indispensable tools in clinical diagnostics, enabling rapid, accurate, and noninvasive analysis of biological samples. Their capacity to translate molecular interactions into measurable optical signals, through fluorescence, absorption, surface plasmon resonance, or Raman scattering, has transformed how diseases are detected, monitored, and managed. By combining advances in photonics, nanotechnology, and biotechnology, modern optical biosensors offer unprecedented speed, sensitivity, and specificity, making them central to the future of precision medicine.

One of the most significant areas of application for optical biosensors is in infectious disease diagnostics. Their ability to detect viral, bacterial, and fungal

Table 2.8 Comparison of optical biosensor types

Type	Detection Principle	Label-Free	Sensitivity	Main Applications
SPR	Surface plasmon resonance	Yes	High	Kinetics, drug binding
Fluorescence	Light emission	No/Yes	Very high	Imaging, multiplex assays
Interferometric	Light interference	Yes	High	Thin-film sensing
Optical fiber	Light transmission	Yes	Moderate–high	In vivo monitoring
Photonic crystal	Refractive index shift	Yes	High	Multiplex detection
Raman (SERS)	Inelastic scattering	Yes	Very high	Structural identification

pathogens with high precision has proven invaluable in both hospital and field settings. During global outbreaks, such as the COVID-19 pandemic, biosensors based on SPR and fluorescence detection were developed to identify viral RNA, proteins, and antibodies with exceptional accuracy and minimal sample preparation. Beyond pandemic response, optical biosensors continue to play a crucial role in diagnosing diseases such as tuberculosis and HIV, where rapid and reliable detection can dramatically improve patient outcomes. Fiber-optic biosensors capable of detecting bacterial endotoxins in real time have shown great promise for early sepsis detection, where immediate intervention is critical. The portability and real-time data output of these systems make them particularly well-suited for point-of-care testing and decentralized diagnostics, especially in low-resource environments.

Cancer diagnostics represent another major field in which optical biosensors have reshaped clinical practice. The early detection of cancer biomarkers, such as carcinoembryonic antigen (CEA), prostate-specific antigen (PSA), CA-125, and HER2, is essential for improving survival rates and treatment efficacy. Optical biosensors, particularly those based on SPR and interferometry, provide label-free, real-time monitoring of tumor-associated molecules at extremely low concentrations [4, 31]. They are also being employed to detect circulating tumor cells in blood, offering a noninvasive method for assessing disease progression and therapeutic response. Fluorescence-based biosensors enable multiplexed detection of genetic mutations and epigenetic changes in tumors, enabling clinicians to perform detailed molecular profiling. This information supports personalized medicine strategies, where treatment decisions are guided by the specific molecular characteristics of a patient's cancer.

In cardiovascular medicine, optical biosensors are used to measure critical biomarkers that indicate heart disease, myocardial injury, or inflammation. Detecting cardiac troponins, C-reactive protein (CRP), and brain natriuretic peptide (BNP) with high sensitivity enables physicians to diagnose acute myocardial infarction within minutes of symptom onset. Microfluidic-integrated optical biosensors allow real-time detection of these biomarkers from a single drop of blood, reducing diagnostic turnaround time in emergency settings. Optical biosensors are also being explored for monitoring lipid levels and cholesterol, supporting long-term cardiovascular health management. The integration of these sensors into wearable or portable devices enables continuous, noninvasive cardiac monitoring, allowing high-risk patients to be tracked outside hospital environments.

Diabetes management has perhaps benefited most visibly from the development of optical biosensors. Traditional glucose monitoring methods rely on finger-prick blood sampling, which can be inconvenient and uncomfortable for patients. In contrast, optical biosensors, using fluorescence, near-infrared absorption, or Raman scattering, enable continuous glucose monitoring in a minimally or noninvasive manner. Wearable sensors integrated into skin patches, smartwatches, or even contact lenses can track glucose levels in real time by measuring glucose concentrations in sweat, tears, or interstitial fluid. This provides a dynamic picture of glycemic control, improving insulin management and overall quality of life for patients with diabetes. These technologies are also being adapted to monitor other metabolic indicators, such as lactate, uric acid, and cholesterol, broadening their application in chronic disease management (Fig. 2.11).

Neurological diseases, which often lack reliable early diagnostic markers, are now being approached through optical biosensing technologies. In neurodegenerative disorders such as Alzheimer's and Parkinson's disease, optical biosensors can detect trace amounts of key biomarkers, such as beta-amyloid peptides, tau proteins, and dopamine, in biological fluids. SPR and fluorescence-based systems allow early-stage detection before clinical symptoms appear, offering opportunities for intervention long before irreversible damage occurs. Optical biosensors are also being developed for real-time monitoring of neurotransmitters and oxidative stress markers, providing valuable insights into disease progression and treatment efficacy. When combined with neuroimaging techniques such as electroencephalography or near-infrared spectroscopy, these sensors support a multimodal diagnostic approach that enhances both sensitivity and diagnostic accuracy (Table 2.9).

The potential of optical biosensors in medicine is vast. They provide not only tools for early disease detection and patient monitoring but also avenues for personalized, preventive healthcare. As technology continues to mature, these sensors are likely to become as commonplace in clinical practice as traditional laboratory assays—bringing rapid, real-time diagnostic capability directly to the point of need.

2.2.5 *Regulatory Considerations*

As optical biosensors become increasingly integrated into medical diagnostics, environmental testing, and food safety monitoring, ensuring their compliance with established regulatory frameworks is essential. These frameworks safeguard public health by ensuring that biosensors are safe, effective, and reliable before they are introduced to the market. Regulatory approval is especially critical for medical applications, where diagnostic accuracy directly affects clinical decisions and patient outcomes.

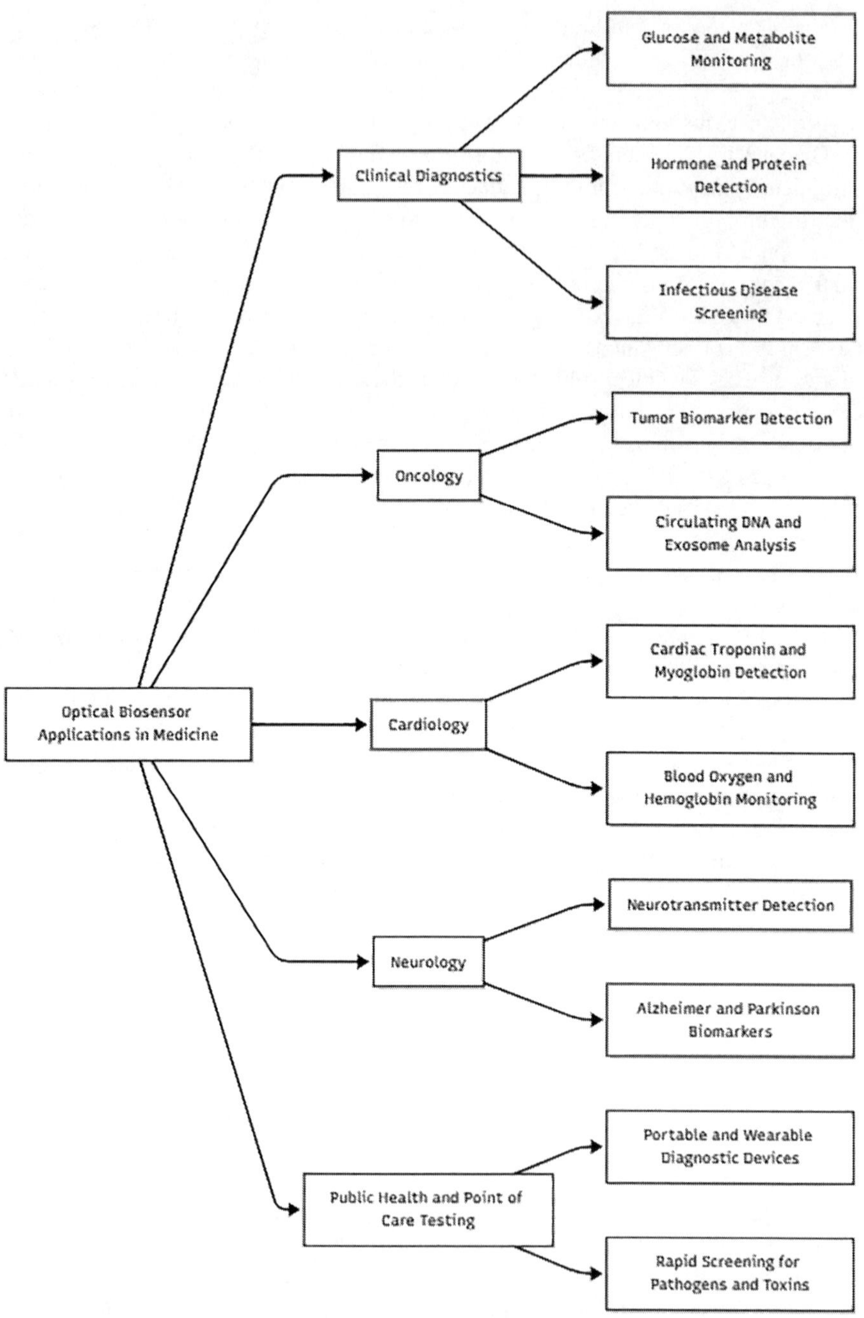

Fig. 2.11 Overview of optical biosensor applications in medicine

Table 2.9 Representative clinical biomarkers detected by optical biosensors

Disease area	Target biomarker	Detection method	Sensor type	Limit of detection	Clinical utility
Infectious	SARS-CoV-2 spike protein	Fluorescence	Fiber-optic	ng/mL	Rapid viral screening
Cancer	PSA, HER2	SPR	Plasmonic chip	pg/mL	Early tumor detection
Cardiovascular	Troponin I, CRP	Interferometric	Lab-on-chip	pg/mL	Myocardial injury
Diabetes	Glucose	NIR, Raman	Wearable optical patch	µM	Continuous monitoring
Neurological	β-amyloid, dopamine	Fluorescence	Microfluidic	ng/mL	Early Alzheimer's diagnosis

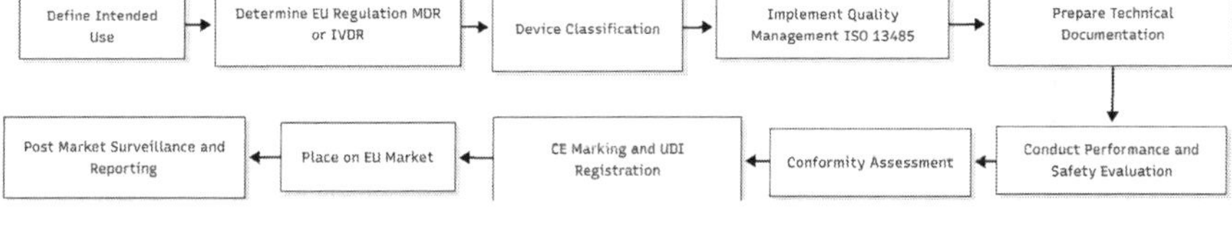

Fig. 2.12 Regulatory approval pathway for optical biosensors

The regulation of optical biosensors is primarily overseen by agencies such as the U.S. FDA, the EMA, and comparable bodies, including Health Canada, the PMDA in Japan, and the notified bodies within the European Union. These organizations classify medical devices based on risk and intended use, dictating the level of testing and documentation required before market approval. High-risk biosensors, such as those used to guide cancer treatment or detect life-threatening infections, undergo far more stringent validation procedures than lower-risk, over-the-counter diagnostic tools.

Optical biosensors are categorized according to risk, mirroring the EU's classification system. Devices are grouped into three main classes: Class I for low-risk devices, Class IIa or IIb for moderate-risk applications, and Class III for high-risk instruments. The classification depends on the sensor's intended purpose, invasiveness, and impact on patient safety. For example, a noninvasive glucose-monitoring biosensor might fall under Class IIa, whereas a biosensor used to guide chemotherapy decisions would typically be classified as Class III due to its clinical significance (Fig. 2.12).

Effective regulation of optical biosensors depends on a balance between encouraging innovation and maintaining rigorous safety standards. As technology continues to advance—particularly through the incorporation of ML, nanomaterials, and wireless data exchange, regulatory agencies are evolving their frameworks to accommodate these innovations. Streamlined approval pathways, clearer software-as a medical-device (SaMD) guidelines, and enhanced post-market monitoring systems are being introduced to ensure that biosensor technologies can reach the market efficiently without compromising patient safety.

Ultimately, regulatory oversight plays a pivotal role in establishing public trust in optical biosensors. By enforcing transparent standards, harmonized international practices, and robust post-market surveillance, regulatory agencies ensure that biosensor technologies continue to deliver accurate, reliable, and ethical outcomes. This regulatory rigor is fundamental not only for clinical acceptance but also for the sustained integration of biosensors into modern healthcare and industry.

2.2.6   Future Perspectives

Optical biosensors are positioned to play an increasingly vital role across medicine, environmental monitoring, biotechnology, and industry. Their ability to provide fast, sensitive, and specific detection of biological and chemical substances has made them essential to modern diagnostics and analytical science. The next generation of optical biosensors will likely be defined by interdisciplinary integration, bringing together advances in nanotechnology, materials science, wearable electronics, artificial intelligence, and wireless communication, to create systems that are more intelligent, autonomous, and accessible than ever before.

A central direction for future development lies in the continued incorporation of nanomaterials and engineered surfaces to improve sensitivity and performance. Nanostructures such as gold nanoparticles, quantum dots, carbon nanotubes, and graphene sheets are already being used to enhance optical signal intensity through effects like localized SPR and SERS [35]. These materials enable biosensors to achieve extraordinarily low detection limits, sometimes reaching femtomolar concentrations. Future devices are expected to utilize hybrid nanomaterials with tunable optical properties, allowing simultaneous detection of multiple analytes in a single platform. For instance, quantum dots with customizable emission spectra could enable multiplexed assays for detecting multiple disease biomarkers simultaneously, while graphene-based photonic films may facilitate ultra-fast, label-free signal transduction.

The emergence of wearable and point-of-care biosensing systems is revolutionizing medical diagnostics. Miniaturized optical biosensors embedded in everyday devices, like smartwatches or phone attachments, are transforming healthcare delivery by enabling real-time monitoring of vital parameters outside hospital settings. These systems use integrated light sources, detectors, and wireless modules to analyze biomarkers and transmit results directly to healthcare providers via mobile applications or cloud platforms [36]. Patients can now perform routine diagnostic tests at home, reducing the need for frequent clinic visits. This accessibility is particularly beneficial for managing chronic conditions, monitoring post-surgical recovery, and providing medical support in remote regions where laboratory infrastructure is limited. Implantable optical biosensors, on the other hand, can provide long-term in vivo monitoring of chronic conditions, drug responses, or postoperative recovery. These innovations reflect a broader shift toward personalized and preventive medicine, where health monitoring becomes an ongoing, interactive process rather than a series of isolated diagnostic events.

AIis set to redefine how biosensors interpret and utilize data. As the complexity of signals from multiplexed and continuous monitoring systems grows, AI and ML algorithms can process vast datasets to identify trends, filter out noise, and build predictive models. Such integration allows biosensors not only to measure but also to analyze and forecast physiological changes in real time. ML models can improve calibration, enhance specificity, and detect anomalies that human operators might overlook. When combined with edge computing, these algorithms can perform real-time analytics directly on the device, reducing reliance on external servers and enabling faster, more secure diagnostics in critical care situations.

The field is also moving toward greater accessibility through point-of-care and low-cost diagnostic devices. Future optical biosensors are expected to become smaller, cheaper, and easier to operate, allowing individuals with minimal technical expertise to perform reliable diagnostic tests at home or in remote environments. Smartphone-integrated biosensors, for example, use the phone's built-in camera and light source to analyze fluorescence, colorimetric, or plasmonic signals [12, 29]. Such systems have the potential to democratize healthcare by bringing laboratory-quality testing to underserved regions, aligning with the World Health Organization's ASSURED principles, Affordable, Sensitive, Specific, User-friendly, Rapid, Equipment-free, and Deliverable to end-users. Portable optical biosensors are already being explored for rapid screening of infectious diseases such as HIV, malaria, and COVID-19, as well as for maternal health monitoring and early cancer detection.

Beyond healthcare, optical biosensors will increasingly impact environmental and industrial sectors. In agriculture, biosensors are being developed to monitor soil nutrients, detect pesticide residues, and identify plant pathogens in real time. In environmental monitoring, they can measure pollutants such as heavy metals, toxins, and microorganisms in air and water. When integrated into drones or autonomous sensor networks, these devices could provide large-scale environmental surveillance, enabling early detection of contamination or ecosystem changes. In industrial biotechnology, optical biosensors are being used to optimize fermentation processes, monitor bioreactor conditions, and ensure the quality and safety of food and pharmaceutical products. These broader applications underline the flexibility and far-reaching potential of optical biosensing technologies.

As optical biosensors become more interconnected and data-driven, regulatory and ethical considerations will grow increasingly important. Devices that store or transmit personal health information must comply with strict data protection and cybersecurity standards. Regulations are evolving to accommodate digital health technologies that combine biosensing, AI, and telemedicine. Agencies such as the FDA and EMA are actively developing adaptive frameworks to accelerate the approval of innovative diagnostic devices while maintaining rigorous safety standards. Future biosensor systems will likely feature end-to-end data encryption, blockchain-based data management, and interoperability with electronic health records to ensure both security and transparency (Fig. 2.13).

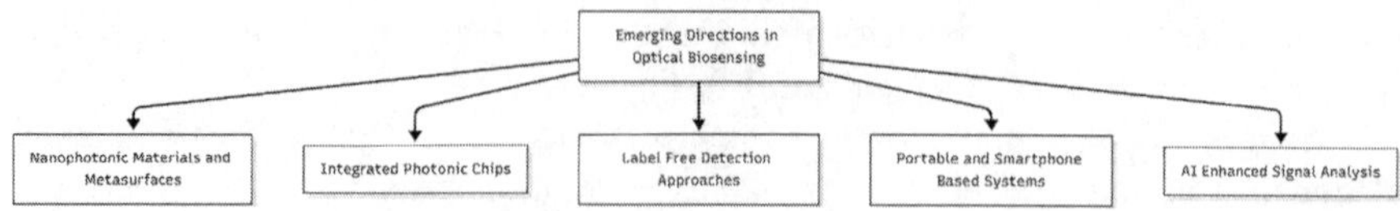

Fig. 2.13 Emerging directions in optical biosensing

Emerging research is expanding the boundaries of optical biosensing in remarkable directions. Developments in holographic biosensors enable three-dimensional imaging of biological processes, while photoacoustic biosensors—combining light excitation with ultrasound detection—enable deep-tissue analysis previously impossible with conventional optics. DNA-based and aptamer-based biosensors are advancing the detection of genetic mutations and real-time gene expression, bringing molecular diagnostics closer to integration with precision therapy [40]. Hybrid systems that merge optical sensing with electrochemical or mechanical transduction methods are also gaining attention for their ability to improve versatility and robustness in complex sample environments.

The long-term vision for optical biosensors is one of full integration into daily life. These technologies are evolving from laboratory instruments into ubiquitous tools embedded in homes, hospitals, and wearable devices. Future biosensors will likely operate as components of digital health ecosystems, connected to cloud-based analytics, virtual healthcare systems, and AI-driven decision-support tools. As they become more affordable and autonomous, they will empower individuals to monitor their own health, manage chronic diseases, and contribute anonymized data to large-scale health research initiatives. Achieving this vision will depend on sustained collaboration between scientists, engineers, clinicians, and policymakers. Continued investment in interdisciplinary research, manufacturing innovation, and harmonized global regulation will be necessary to ensure that optical biosensors reach their full potential. As they continue to evolve, these devices are poised to transform not only how diseases are detected and managed but also how society approaches wellness, sustainability, and environmental stewardship. The future of optical biosensing thus represents a convergence of technology and humanity, where light becomes a universal language for understanding and improving life itself.

2.3 Impedance Biosensors

Electrochemical impedance spectroscopy is a powerful analytical technique that enables the detailed examination of the kinetic and transport properties of electrochemical systems within a single experimental framework. By applying an alternating current (AC) signal to an electrochemical cell and measuring the resulting current response, EIS provides insight into a system's rate constants, diffusion coefficients, and other essential parameters. Unlike techniques that rely on nonlinear responses, such as cyclic voltammetry, EIS operates within the linear range of electrical excitation, allowing the system to be described mathematically using ordinary differential equations. For this reason, EIS is especially effective when the applied voltage remains below approximately 25 mV at room temperature, ensuring that the system behaves linearly and that charge transfer reactions can be treated as proportional to the applied potential.

This linearity requirement defines the conditions under which impedance measurements can yield reliable data. When these parameters are satisfied, certain system characteristics, such as the ohmic resistance of an electrolyte or the thickness of a passivating film on an electrode, can remain constant over a wide range of experimental conditions [41]. Once determined, these values can be used to model electrochemical behavior under more complex or variable situations.

A defining feature of impedance spectroscopy is that it transforms time-domain signals into the frequency domain, enabling researchers to calculate impedance as a complex function of voltage and current. Impedance is inherently a complex quantity that represents both the resistive and reactive components of the system's response. By examining how impedance varies with frequency, an impedance spectrum is obtained, providing a unique "fingerprint" of the electrochemical processes occurring at the electrode interface. EIS shares methodological similarities with other linear-excitation electrochemical techniques, such as potential-step or current-step methods, but its analytical strength lies in the frequency-dependent characterization of system behavior. Through frequency-domain analysis, EIS can separate overlapping physical and chemical processes that would otherwise be indistinguishable in the time domain. This capability allows researchers to isolate contributions from charge transfer, diffusion, adsorption, and double-layer capacitance within a single experiment.

The impedance spectrum can be interpreted using equivalent circuit models, in which the electrochemical system is represented by discrete electrical elements such as resistors, capacitors, and inductors. These models serve as practical approximations that help simplify complex electrochemical behavior into interpretable components. By fitting experimental data to such models, it becomes possible to derive quantitative parameters that describe interfacial phenomena, reaction kinetics, and transport processes (Table 2.10).

Table 2.10 Comparison between EIS and other electrochemical techniques

Technique	Excitation type	Response measured	Frequency dependence	Key output	Main application
Cyclic voltammetry	Linear potential sweep	Current	No	Redox peaks	Kinetics
Chronoamperometry	Step potential	Current vs. time	No	Decay curves	Diffusion
EIS	Sinusoidal AC	Voltage and current	Yes	Impedance spectra	Interface characterization

Because impedance models are generally simpler in the frequency domain than in the time domain, computational analysis becomes more efficient and accurate. Modern computing tools enable rapid optimization of model parameters, even for intricate systems involving multiple coupled reactions. Consequently, EIS has become indispensable in the study of corrosion mechanisms, electrode kinetics, energy storage devices, and biosensors [42]. Its versatility lies in its ability to simultaneously probe both the thermodynamic and kinetic properties of a system, making it one of the most comprehensive electrochemical characterization methods available today.

2.3.1 History

The development of EIS can be traced back to the late nineteenth century, when foundational work in electrical theory began shaping the study of electrochemical systems. The conceptual groundwork was laid by Oliver Heaviside through his formulation of Linear Systems Theory, which described how electrical systems respond to linear excitations. Around the same period, Walther Nernst and later Erich Warburg extended these ideas to electrochemistry. Warburg introduced the concept of impedance as a function describing diffusion-controlled processes, and his model, now known as the Warburg impedance, remains a cornerstone of modern electrochemical analysis.

In the early twentieth century, EIS found practical use in studies of metal electrodes, particularly through the use of reactive bridges to measure the capacitance of ideally polarizable surfaces such as mercury. These early experiments contributed to the first models of the electrified interface, where charge separation occurs between an electrode and an electrolyte [43]. However, it was not until the mid-twentieth century that the technique began to evolve into a more refined and accessible analytical tool.

A major turning point came with the invention of the potentiostat in the 1940s, which allowed for precise control of electrode potentials during electrochemical measurements. This innovation provided the stability needed to conduct frequency-dependent experiments and sparked a surge of interest in electrochemical kinetics and corrosion research. By the 1970s, the introduction of frequency response analyzers further advanced EIS by enabling accurate impedance measurements across a wide range of frequencies, including very low-frequency domains critical for studying slow interfacial processes.

As instrumentation improved, EIS was increasingly applied to a variety of materials and systems, from solid and liquid conductors to polymers, coatings, and biological interfaces. Researchers began using impedance data to elucidate complex reaction mechanisms, monitor passivation phenomena, and characterize ionic and electronic conduction in emerging materials. The method's ability to separate and quantify multiple processes occurring simultaneously—such as charge transfer, diffusion, and adsorption, made it particularly valuable for both fundamental studies and applied research.

Historically, the analytical interpretation of EIS data relied on human pattern recognition through visual inspection of Nyquist or Bode plots. However, as datasets grew in complexity, there was a growing need for computational approaches capable of automating the identification of reaction mechanisms. Recent discussions in the field have proposed that integrating artificial intelligence, particularly artificial neural networks, could transform EIS analysis by enabling automated pattern recognition and model fitting. This would require establishing large libraries of theoretical impedance spectra associated with known reaction mechanisms, forming the basis for data-driven interpretation.

Over more than a century of development, EIS has evolved from a theoretical construct into a versatile experimental method used across disciplines [44]. Its integration with modern electronics, computational modeling, and ML continues to expand its reach, solidifying its role as one of the most insightful tools for probing electrochemical and biosensing systems (Fig. 2.14).

2.3.2 Technical Characteristics

EIS biosensors are sophisticated analytical systems that characterize and quantify biochemical interactions via electrical measurements. Their architecture combines several essential components that work together to convert molecular recognition events into measurable impedance signals. These components include the electrodes, biorecognition layer, electrolyte medium, and supporting electronic instrumentation. The performance of an EIS biosensor depends on the precision of its hardware setup, the quality of signal acquisition, and the efficiency of data analysis and interpretation (Table 2.11).

Hardware
The construction of an EIS biosensor involves a standard three-electrode configuration consisting of a working electrode, a reference electrode, and a counter electrode. The working electrode, often made from screen-printed carbon (SPCE) or glassy carbon (GCE), is the central site where the biorecognition process occurs. The reference electrode, commonly silver/silver chloride (Ag/AgCl), provides a stable potential against which all measurements are made, while the platinum

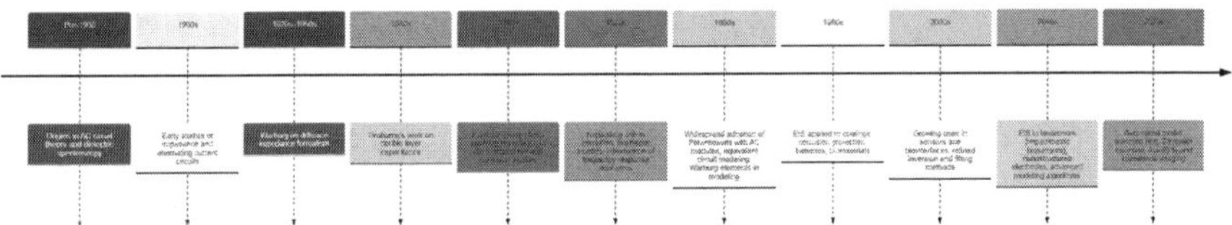

Fig. 2.14 Timeline of EIS development and milestones

Table 2.11 Common electrode materials and their properties in EIS biosensors

Material	Conductivity	Biocompatibility	Common modification	Application
Gold	High	Excellent	Thiol SAMs, AuNPs	Enzyme/antibody immobilization
Carbon	Moderate	Good	CNTs, graphene	DNA sensors
Platinum	High	Excellent	Polymer films	Catalytic reactions
ITO	Moderate	Transparent	Metal oxides	Optical–electrochemical hybrids

counter electrode completes the circuit by allowing current to flow through the electrolyte solution.

The electrolyte typically consists of phosphate-buffered saline (PBS) at physiological pH, ensuring ionic conductivity and chemical stability during measurements [45]. Depending on the specific application, the working electrode surface is modified to enhance conductivity and immobilize biorecognition elements such as enzymes, antibodies, or aptamers. Surface modifications frequently include the deposition of nanomaterials, such as gold nanoparticles, carbon nanotubes, or graphene derivatives, to increase the electroactive surface area and facilitate electron transfer.

Immobilization of biological elements is achieved through chemical cross-linking or covalent attachment using agents such as glutaraldehyde or EDC/NHS (1-ethyl-3-(3-dimethylaminopropyl) carbodiimide and N-hydroxysuccinimide). These linkers ensure stable and oriented attachment of biomolecules without significantly impairing their biological activity. For impedance measurements, a redox probe such as ferricyanide/ferrocyanide ($[Fe(CN)_6]^{3-/4-}$) is often used to mediate electron transfer between the electrode surface and the analyte.

The hardware setup is connected to an electrochemical workstation, such as those produced by Autolab or CH Instruments, capable of applying AC voltages across a range of frequencies and recording the resulting current responses. The measurement typically spans frequencies between 0.1 Hz and 100 kHz, with an applied AC amplitude of 5–10 mV to maintain system linearity. This range captures both fast interfacial processes, such as charge transfer, and slower diffusion-controlled reactions.

Software

The software component is integral to both controlling the experiment and interpreting impedance data. Programs such as NOVA and ZView are commonly employed to design frequency sweeps, collect data, and fit results to equivalent circuit models. The Randles circuit is the most frequently used model, representing the electrochemical interface through a combination of resistive and capacitive elements. Within this framework, key parameters, including solution resistance (Rs), charge transfer resistance (Rct), and double-layer capacitance (Cdl), are extracted.

The biosensor is calibrated by measuring impedance changes at varying analyte concentrations and plotting the data to establish a calibration curve. The slope of this curve indicates sensitivity, while the limit of detection (LOD), linear dynamic range, and selectivity are used to assess performance [46]. Automated fitting routines within the analysis software provide numerical values for each circuit parameter, which can then be correlated with biochemical interactions occurring at the electrode surface. Advanced data processing involves noise filtering, baseline correction, and phase angle analysis to separate contributions from different electrochemical phenomena. The software also enables real-time monitoring and modeling, allowing observation of binding events or enzymatic reactions as they occur. Through these analytical capabilities, impedance biosensors can achieve high levels of reproducibility, stability, and quantitative accuracy.

The combination of well-engineered hardware and advanced analytical software gives EIS biosensors their versatility and precision. They can detect a wide range of biological and chemical analytes with high sensitivity and selectivity, even in complex sample matrices. As instrumentation continues to evolve—particularly with the integration of automation, miniaturization, and wireless communication, EIS-based systems are becoming increasingly adaptable for point-of-care diagnostics and field applications.

The principle of EIS is based on the concept that, when an electrochemical reaction occurs at an electrode–electrolyte interface, it involves both charge-transfer and mass-transport processes that contribute to the system's overall impedance. By analyzing how these processes respond to sinusoidal perturbations, researchers can derive critical information about reaction kinetics, diffusion, and interfacial properties. At its core, EIS measures the opposition of a system to an applied AC signal, expressed as impedance, a complex quantity combining both resistance and reactance. The system's response is evaluated over a frequency range to produce an impedance profile that reflects the dynamic interactions within the electrochemical cell [47]. High-frequency signals typically probe processes associated with the double-layer capacitance and solution resistance, whereas low-frequency signals reveal slower phenomena such as charge transfer reactions, diffusion, and adsorption. When an electrochemical reaction occurs, the electrode surface participates in two simultaneous processes: faradaic and non-faradaic. Faradaic processes involve actual charge transfer across the interface as electrons are exchanged during oxidation or reduction reactions, such as the transformation of an oxidized species (O) into its reduced form (R). Non-faradaic processes, in contrast, arise from the charging and discharging of the electrical double layer, a capacitive phenomenon that does not involve any chemical change but influences the overall impedance response.

To interpret these complex interfacial events, EIS data are often modeled using electrical equivalent circuits (EECs). The most common of these models is the Randles circuit, which represents the electrochemical interface as a network of resistors, capacitors, and sometimes diffusional elements known as Warburg impedances. Each circuit component corresponds to a specific physical process: the solution resistance (Rs) accounts for ion transport through the electrolyte; the double-layer capacitance (Cdl) represents charge accumulation at the interface; the charge transfer resistance (Rct) reflects the kinetic barrier for electron transfer; and the Warburg impedance (Zw) models diffusion of reactants and products near the electrode surface (Fig. 2.15).

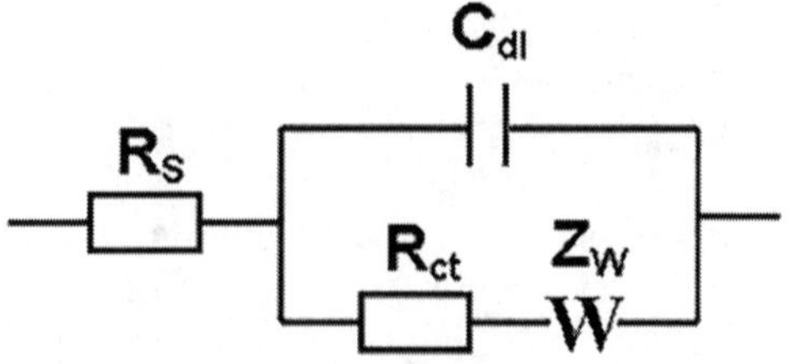

Fig. 2.15 Randles circuit model (https://commons.wikimedia.org/wiki/File:Randles_circuit.png)

During an EIS experiment, the applied AC signal is intentionally small—usually between 5 and 10 mV—to maintain linear system behavior and prevent perturbation of the equilibrium state. The excitation frequency is systematically varied from high to low values, allowing the observation of processes with different characteristic time constants. The resulting impedance data are then plotted on Nyquist or Bode diagrams, which visualize the real and imaginary components of impedance. These plots reveal distinctive patterns, such as semicircular arcs or linear tails, that correspond to specific electrochemical mechanisms.

One of the most significant advantages of EIS is its ability to extract comprehensive kinetic parameters from a single experimental run. Unlike time-domain techniques, which often require multiple experiments to study different aspects of system behavior, EIS provides information on rate constants, diffusion coefficients, and interfacial capacitances in one analysis. Furthermore, because impedance spectra are obtained in the frequency domain, the method allows for mathematical separation of overlapping processes that occur simultaneously, such as charge transfer and mass transport, something that would be extremely difficult to achieve using conventional voltammetric or amperometric methods. The charge-transfer resistance, often denoted Rct, is a key parameter for evaluating biosensor performance because it is directly influenced by the binding of target analytes to the biorecognition layer. When analyte molecules bind to immobilized biomolecules, such as enzymes, antibodies, or aptamers, they alter the interfacial structure and, consequently, the impedance profile. A higher Rct typically indicates increased surface blockage due to successful binding, whereas a lower Rct suggests enhanced electron transfer through conductive nanomaterials or surface modifications [48]. Because of its high sensitivity, EIS is particularly effective for monitoring biomolecular interactions at extremely low analyte concentrations, often without the need for labeling or complex sample preparation. It also provides insights into the condition of electrode surfaces, including the formation of passivating films, corrosion layers, and biofouling (Table 2.12).

In essence, EIS provides a frequency-resolved view of the processes governing electrochemical reactions. By combining precise instrumentation with theoretical modeling, EIS enables researchers to dissect complex interfacial phenomena into measurable parameters that describe charge transfer, capacitance, and diffusion. This makes it an indispensable technique not only for biosensing but also for corrosion studies, battery analysis, and material characterization.

Table 2.12 Interpretation of EIS parameters in biosensing

Parameter	Symbol	Physical meaning	Affected by	Indicates
Solution resistance	Rs	Electrolyte conductivity	Ionic strength	Medium composition
Charge-transfer resistance	Rct	Electron transfer barrier	Analyte binding	Sensor sensitivity
Double-layer capacitance	Cdl	Surface charge storage	Surface modification	Interface structure
Warburg impedance	Zw	Diffusion of ions	Concentration gradients	Mass transport

2.3.3   Types of Devices

Electrochemical biosensors are widely recognized for their precision, adaptability, and suitability across diverse analytical applications. Among these, impedance-based biosensors stand out for their exceptional sensitivity in detecting biochemical events such as DNA hybridization, antigen–antibody binding, enzyme activity, and drug–receptor interactions. These sensors quantify changes in electrical properties, most commonly potential, current, or impedance, resulting from molecular recognition at the electrode interface. The measurable electrical response is proportional to the concentration of the electroactive species, allowing for accurate quantification of the analyte in complex biological or environmental samples. Compared to optical biosensors, electrochemical systems offer several advantages, including greater stability, faster response times, and reduced susceptibility to environmental factors such as temperature and light. Their operation requires simpler instrumentation, and their electrical signals can be easily processed, making them ideal for miniaturized and portable detection platforms. Owing to these benefits, electrochemical methods have become the preferred choice for biosensing applications that demand high sensitivity and rapid, real-time measurements. Electrochemical biosensors are generally classified according to the specific electrical parameter they measure. The four principal categories include conductometric, potentiometric, amperometric, and impedimetric biosensors. Each type operates on distinct electrochemical principles, targeting different aspects of electron flow, ionic movement, or potential changes at the sensor surface [49].

Impedimetric biosensors monitor changes in the impedance of an electrochemical system as molecular interactions occur at the sensor surface. When an analyte binds to its corresponding recognition element, the resulting modification of the electrode interface alters its charge transfer resistance and capacitance. These variations can be precisely measured using EIS, providing a highly sensitive, label-free detection method. Impedimetric biosensors are particularly effective for identifying microorganisms, toxins, and biomarkers in medical, environmental, and food samples. Their ability to perform real-time monitoring without requiring fluorescent or radioactive labels makes them a preferred option in modern biosensing research and diagnostics (Table 2.13).

Table 2.13 Comparison among electrochemical biosensor types

Type	Measured quantity	Signal type	Advantages	Limitations	Example application
Conductometric	Conductivity	Current flow	Simple setup	Low S/N ratio	Ion detection
Potentiometric	Potential difference	Voltage	High selectivity	Limited sensitivity	pH sensors
Amperometric	Current	Electron transfer	Fast, sensitive	Requires redox species	Glucose sensors
Impedimetric	Impedance	Complex resistance	Label-free, real-time	Requires modeling	Biomarker detection

Electrochemical impedance biosensors are available in multiple configurations, each designed for specific analytical, clinical, or field-based applications. Their diversity reflects the range of operational needs—from laboratory research requiring high-precision instrumentation to portable and wearable systems tailored for real-time monitoring. The classification of these devices is generally based on their level of integration, portability, and intended application environment (Fig. 2.16).

Bench-top systems represent the most advanced and high-precision category of EIS biosensors. These laboratory-grade instruments combine a potentiostat with impedance measurement capabilities and are typically used for fundamental electrochemical research, materials characterization, and calibration of prototype sensors. They offer exceptional sensitivity and control, enabling detailed analysis of interfacial processes over a broad frequency range. Bench-top systems are essential for developing and validating new biosensor designs before transitioning to portable or commercial formats.

Portable handheld devices have been developed to bring the advantages of impedance-based analysis beyond the laboratory setting. These compact systems are powered by batteries and feature integrated electronics for data acquisition and basic signal processing. They are particularly valuable for point-of-care diagnostics and rapid testing in clinical or remote environments. User-friendly interfaces and automated calibration routines allow operation without specialized training, making them ideal for healthcare professionals and field technicians alike.

Wearable biosensors represent a rapidly growing segment of electrochemical impedance technology. These flexible, lightweight devices are designed to be integrated into textiles, skin patches, or accessories to continuously monitor biomarkers such as glucose, lactate, or electrolytes in sweat or interstitial fluid [50]. The incorporation of conductive polymers and graphene-based materials enhances signal stability while maintaining comfort and flexibility. Wearable EIS biosensors enable real-time health monitoring and personalized medical care by transmitting data wirelessly to smartphones or cloud-based systems.

Microfluidic biosensors, often referred to as lab-on-a-chip systems, combine sample handling, sensing, and analysis within a compact platform. These devices use microchannels to precisely control fluid flow and ensure efficient interaction between the analyte and the sensor surface. The integration of EIS technology into microfluidic devices enables rapid detection with minimal sample volume, high

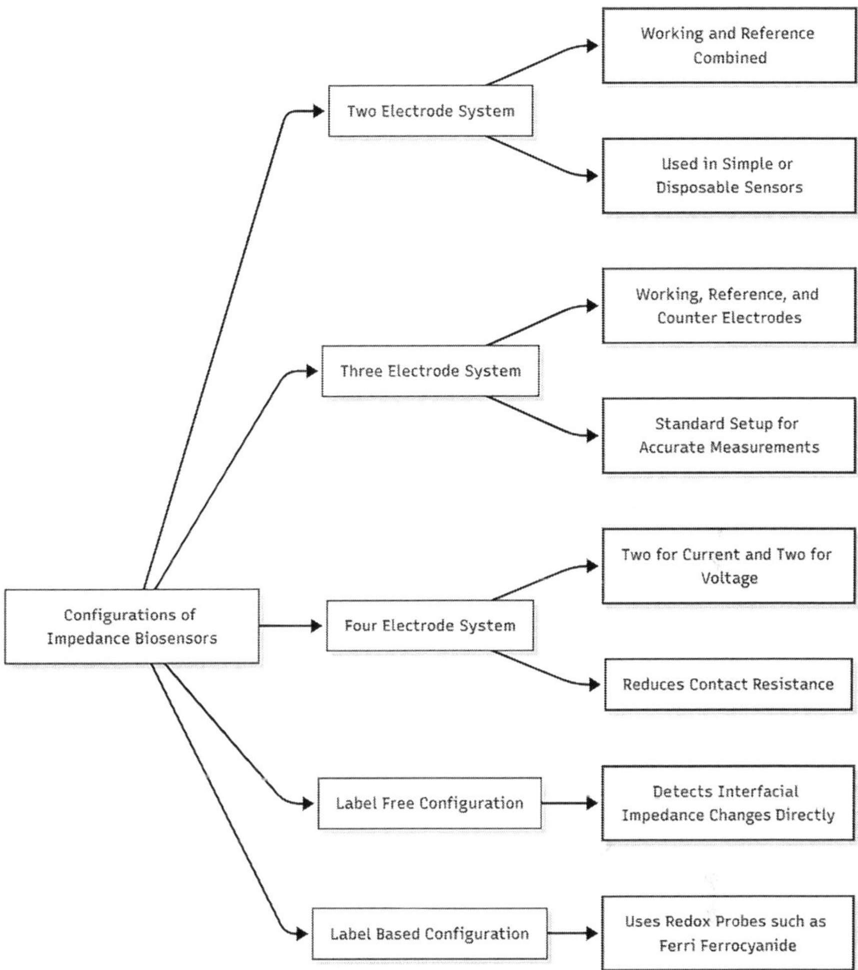

Fig. 2.16 Configurations of impedance biosensors

throughput, and reduced contamination risk. They are particularly useful for diagnostic applications requiring multiplexed testing or small-scale biological assays, such as monitoring pathogens or biomarkers in complex fluids.

Smartphone-integrated biosensors bridge the gap between advanced instrumentation and consumer accessibility. These systems connect to smartphones via Bluetooth, NFC, or USB interfaces, using the phone's processing power and display for data visualization. Miniaturized electrodes and microchips perform the impedance measurements, while companion mobile applications handle calibration, signal analysis, and data storage [51]. The convenience and portability of smartphone-based biosensors make them suitable for home diagnostics, environmental testing, and telemedicine applications.

Implantable biosensors represent the most advanced and specialized category, designed for continuous in vivo monitoring of physiological parameters. These miniaturized systems can operate for long periods within biological tissues, providing real-time insights into metabolic activity, drug response, and disease progression. Their development requires careful consideration of biocompatibility, stability, and wireless data transmission. Although still in the early stages of clinical adoption, implantable EIS biosensors hold great promise for future medical applications, particularly in chronic disease management and personalized therapeutics.

2.3.4 Clinical Applications

The application of electrochemical biosensors has expanded dramatically over the past two decades, driven by the need for rapid, reliable, and cost-effective analytical tools across medicine, environmental science, food safety, and biotechnology. Traditional laboratory-based analysis often involves sending samples to centralized facilities, where they are tested using complex, time-consuming methods that require skilled personnel and expensive instrumentation. While such methods deliver high precision, their logistical and financial demands limit their accessibility. In contrast, biosensor technology offers an efficient alternative, enabling on-site, real-time analysis without compromising sensitivity or accuracy. This shift from conventional testing to decentralized diagnostics has fueled the remarkable growth of biosensor research and development. Electrochemical biosensors, including those based on impedance measurements, have become indispensable for environmental monitoring, disease diagnostics, drug discovery, and food quality control. Their adaptability, low power requirements, and straightforward electrical readouts make them suitable for both laboratory and field settings. The following sections outline key domains where EIS biosensors have demonstrated significant impact, emphasizing medical applications and selected real-world case studies (Fig. 2.17).

The medical field has benefited enormously from advances in biosensor technology. These devices exploit molecular interactions at the sensor surface to detect and quantify biological markers associated with various diseases. Applications include cancer diagnosis, cardiovascular monitoring, diabetes management, and infectious disease detection [52]. Because EIS biosensors can operate without labeling agents, they offer real-time detection while minimizing preparation time and cost.

In **cancer research** and **clinical oncology,** biosensors are being used to identify tumor biomarkers such as HER2, PSA, and CEA, which are indicative of specific

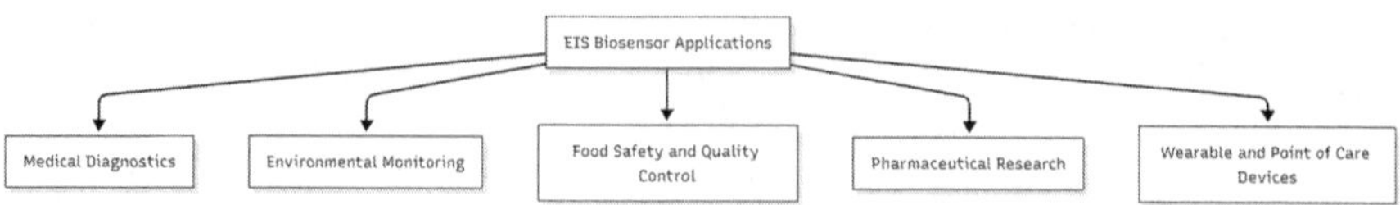

Fig. 2.17 Schematic representation of EIS biosensor applications

cancer types and disease stages. By detecting these markers in blood or serum samples, EIS-based biosensors allow early diagnosis and continuous monitoring of treatment effectiveness. Their high sensitivity enables the detection of biomolecules at extremely low concentrations, which is essential for identifying malignancies before they progress to advanced stages. Moreover, multiplexed detection enables comprehensive molecular profiling for personalized cancer therapy.

Cardiovascular diseases remain a leading cause of mortality worldwide, underscoring the importance of early and accurate biomarker detection. Electrochemical biosensors provide a fast and efficient means of measuring cardiac indicators such as troponins, C-reactive protein (CRP), and brain natriuretic peptide (BNP). The rapid response of impedance-based devices makes them invaluable in emergency medicine, where timely diagnosis can significantly affect patient outcomes. Their portability also supports bedside and ambulatory testing, thereby improving patient management and enabling faster decision-making.

In the context of **diabetes care**, biosensors have revolutionized glucose monitoring. EIS and amperometric biosensors enable continuous or semi-continuous glucose detection via enzymatic reactions catalyzed by glucose oxidase [53]. Recent advances have introduced wearable and noninvasive sensors capable of detecting glucose in sweat, saliva, or interstitial fluid, eliminating the discomfort associated with traditional finger-prick testing. These innovations are transforming diabetes management by providing real-time feedback that enables better glycemic control and the prevention of complications.

Neurological and infectious diseases have also seen growing use of EIS biosensors. In neurodegenerative disorders such as Alzheimer's and Parkinson's, sensors capable of detecting biomarkers like tau and beta-amyloid proteins are being developed for early diagnosis and monitoring of disease progression. In infectious disease diagnostics, electrochemical biosensors have proven highly effective for detecting bacterial and viral pathogens—including *E. coli*, *Salmonella*, and SARS-CoV-2—due to their rapid response, low detection limits, and minimal sample processing requirements.

2.3.5 *Regulatory Considerations*

All biosensors, including impedimetric, intended for medical diagnostics are generally classified as medical devices and fall under the jurisdiction of national and international regulatory agencies. In the European Union, these devices are governed by the Medical Device Regulation (MDR 2017/745), which outlines strict requirements for design validation, clinical evaluation, and post-market surveillance. In the United States, the FDA regulates medical biosensors under Title 21 of the Code of Federal Regulations. Depending on their intended purpose and associated risk, biosensors may fall into Class I, II, or III, with Class III requiring the most rigorous premarket approval process.

Validation and performance assessment form the foundation of the regulatory approval process. Manufacturers must provide evidence of analytical accuracy, precision, sensitivity, specificity, linear range, reproducibility, and limit of detection (LOD). International standards such as ISO 13485, which governs quality management systems for medical devices, and ISO 15197, which applies to glucose monitoring systems, provide frameworks for ensuring that biosensors meet consistent performance criteria [54]. These standards also address component traceability, documentation practices, and risk management throughout the device's life cycle.

Another essential consideration is biocompatibility, particularly for biosensors that come into direct contact with biological tissues or fluids. The materials used must not elicit cytotoxic, allergenic, or inflammatory responses. Compliance with ISO 10993, which covers the biological evaluation of medical devices, ensures that biosensors meet accepted biocompatibility standards. Devices containing electrical components must also comply with IEC 60601, which governs the safety and electromagnetic compatibility of medical electrical equipment. This standard ensures that biosensors do not interfere with other electronic medical instruments and remain safe under various environmental and operational conditions.

Labeling and documentation requirements are equally critical. Manufacturers must provide comprehensive instructions for use, warnings, and risk assessments. A technical file, or design dossier, is required as part of the regulatory submission and must include detailed information on the device's composition, intended function, performance data, and quality assurance procedures. Transparent labeling and accurate information enable healthcare professionals and users to operate the biosensor safely and effectively (Fig. 2.18).

Clinical evaluation is often necessary to demonstrate that a biosensor performs as intended in real-world conditions. For diagnostic devices, clinical studies are used to confirm that laboratory performance translates into reliable clinical outcomes. These studies assess both the accuracy of results and their reproducibility across diverse patient populations. In high-risk applications or when novel biomarkers are involved, formal clinical trials may be mandated before market authorization is granted.

After approval, biosensors enter the post-market phase, where manufacturers are required to maintain continuous surveillance of device performance. This includes monitoring for adverse events, device malfunctions, and user-reported issues. Regular safety and performance updates must be submitted to regulatory authorities to ensure ongoing compliance. Post-market obligations are critical for identifying potential risks that may only become apparent after widespread use and for ensuring that corrective actions are implemented promptly.

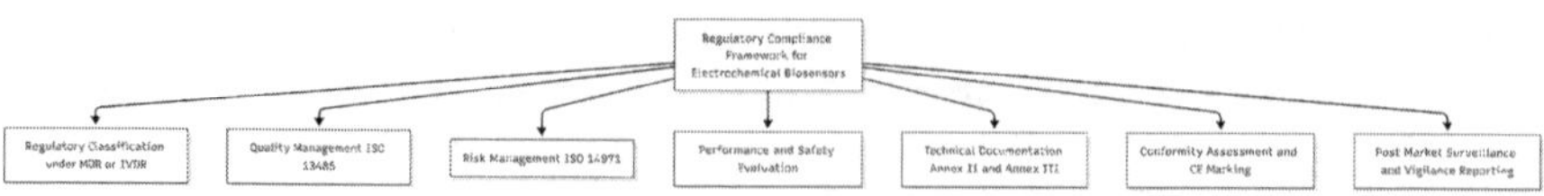

Fig. 2.18 Regulatory compliance framework for electrochemical biosensors

2.3.6 Future Perspectives

EIS-based biosensors are emerging as one of the most promising technologies for rapid, sensitive, and label-free detection across medical, environmental, and industrial fields. As research progresses, several technological and scientific trends are shaping the future of these systems, driving their transition from laboratory instruments to practical, real-world diagnostic tools. One of the most significant directions for advancement lies in miniaturization and portability. The continuous development of microfabrication, flexible electronics, and lab-on-a-chip technologies is enabling the construction of smaller, more versatile biosensors capable of operating outside traditional laboratory settings. By integrating EIS with microfluidic channels and portable electronics, researchers are creating compact systems that perform precise, real-time analyses with minimal sample volumes [55]. These platforms are particularly well-suited for point-of-care diagnostics, where accessibility, affordability, and rapid results are essential. Wearable and implantable formats are also gaining traction, offering continuous monitoring of biomarkers in biological fluids such as sweat, saliva, or interstitial fluid.

The expansion of point-of-care applications is another major focus. Impedance-based biosensors are ideal for decentralized testing because they require low power, provide quick readouts, and can operate with minimal user intervention. Integration with smartphones and wireless data transmission technologies is transforming these devices into connected diagnostic tools that can transmit data instantly to healthcare providers. Such innovations are expected to enhance disease surveillance, improve patient management, and reduce dependence on centralized laboratories, particularly in low-resource or remote settings.

Another transformative trend involves nanomaterial-enhanced sensitivity. The incorporation of advanced nanostructures—such as graphene, carbon nanotubes, metal–organic frameworks, and gold nanoparticles—has revolutionized the performance of EIS biosensors. These materials increase the electroactive surface area, facilitate faster electron transfer, and enhance the immobilization of biological molecules, thereby improving sensitivity and lowering detection limits. Future research is likely to focus on the rational design of hybrid nanocomposites that combine the conductivity of metals, the stability of carbon materials, and the selectivity of biological receptors. Such innovations could allow detection of analytes at femtomolar or even attomolar levels, expanding the range of detectable biomarkers.

The integration of AI and data analytics into biosensing platforms is also redefining how impedance data are interpreted and applied. ML algorithms can identify patterns in complex impedance spectra, automate signal interpretation, and predict analyte concentrations with remarkable accuracy. These algorithms are particularly useful for multiplexed sensing systems, which detect multiple analytes simultaneously, yielding multidimensional data. AI-based models not only improve biosensor accuracy but also enable adaptive calibration, anomaly detection, and real-time decision-making. In the future, edge computing technologies will enable such data processing directly within the biosensor device, minimizing reliance on cloud infrastructure and improving response times for critical diagnostics.

Multiplexed and intelligent sensing is another growing research frontier. Future EIS biosensors are expected to incorporate multiple sensing sites or microelectrode arrays to detect multiple biomarkers in parallel. Combined with embedded microprocessors and AI-driven algorithms, these systems could perform complex diagnostic assessments, such as detecting multiple pathogens in a single test or monitoring entire metabolic profiles in real time [56]. This approach aligns closely with the global trend toward personalized and precision medicine, where healthcare decisions are tailored to an individual's specific biochemical and physiological state.

Regulatory and commercial challenges remain central to the widespread adoption of EIS biosensors. Streamlining validation procedures, establishing standardized testing protocols, and harmonizing international regulations will be essential for accelerating market entry. At the same time, ensuring data security and patient privacy will become increasingly important as biosensors become connected to digital health networks. Future regulatory frameworks are expected to evolve in parallel with technological progress, incorporating cybersecurity standards, software validation procedures, and ethical guidelines for AI-assisted diagnostics.

Sustainability is also emerging as a key design principle in biosensor development. The creation of eco-friendly and disposable sensing platforms using biodegradable polymers, paper-based substrates, or recyclable materials can reduce environmental impact while maintaining affordability. These sustainable sensors are particularly valuable for large-scale screening programs and environmental applications, where single-use devices are often preferred (Table 2.14).

In addition to healthcare and diagnostics, future EIS biosensors are expected to play an increasingly important role in environmental and industrial monitoring. In agriculture, they may be used to detect pesticide residues, pathogens, and soil nutrients, thereby supporting safer, more sustainable food production. In bioprocessing and pharmaceutical manufacturing, integrated biosensors will provide continuous quality control by monitoring fermentation parameters, nutrient levels, and contamination in real time [57]. Environmental biosensors capable of detecting

Table 2.14 Future research trends and expected impacts

Innovation area	Description	Expected outcome	Application example
Nanomaterials	Hybrid AuNP-graphene composites	Ultra-low detection limits	Cancer biomarkers
AI-assisted modeling	ML for EIS spectra	Automated interpretation	Multiplex analysis
Miniaturization	Flexible, microfluidic integration	Portable diagnostics	Point-of-care
Sustainability	Paper-based or biodegradable sensors	Eco-friendly disposal	Field testing
Implantable EIS	Biocompatible real-time monitoring	Continuous health tracking	Chronic diseases

pollutants such as heavy metals, toxins, and microbial contaminants in air or water will contribute to more effective public health protection and ecosystem management.

2.4   Acoustic and Piezoelectric Biosensors

Biosensors have become essential analytical tools in diagnostics, environmental monitoring, and biological research due to the growing demand for rapid, precise, and noninvasive detection methods. They bridge the gap between biological recognition and signal transduction, providing real-time insights into molecular interactions and physiological changes. Among the various biosensing platforms available, acoustic and piezoelectric biosensors stand out for their high sensitivity, ability to operate without labeling agents, and suitability for continuous monitoring [58]. These qualities make them ideal for studying complex biochemical systems under natural or physiological conditions (Fig. 2.19).

Two of the most prominent types of acoustic biosensors are the **Quartz Crystal Microbalance (QCM) and Surface Acoustic Wave (SAW)** sensors. Both rely on the piezoelectric effect, a phenomenon in which mechanical stress applied to a piezoelectric crystal generates an electric charge, or conversely, an electric field induces mechanical deformation. In practice, these sensors detect alterations in wave properties, such as resonance frequency, propagation velocity, or energy dissipation, that occur when biological molecules bind to their surfaces. The resulting signal variations provide quantitative information about the binding events and the physical properties of the adsorbed layer. The exceptional sensitivity of QCM and SAW sensors to mass and viscoelastic changes makes them valuable for studying biomolecular interactions involving proteins, nucleic acids, pathogens, and other biologically relevant compounds. Their capability to measure nanoscale mass variations in real time, without the need for fluorescent or radioactive labeling, gives them a distinct advantage over many optical or electrochemical techniques. These sensors are also well-suited for applications in molecular diagnostics, pharmacological screening, and environmental biosurveillance, where speed and accuracy are critical.

Recent developments have further enhanced their potential by integrating QCM and SAW technologies with microfluidic systems. Such integration enables precise control of liquid handling, sample conditioning, and analyte delivery, allowing multiplexed analysis and improved reproducibility. The addition of microfluidics also supports sensor miniaturization, reduces reagent consumption, and facilitates automation [59]. Combined with advances in nanomaterials, surface functionalization,

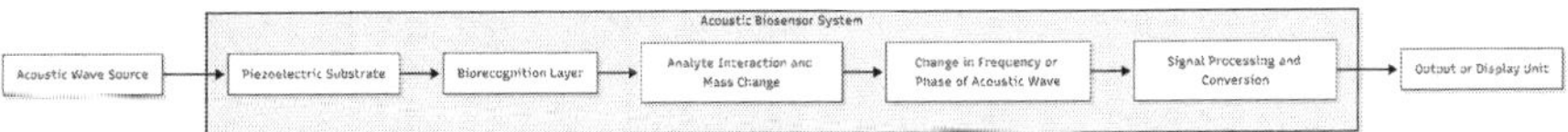

Fig. 2.19 General architecture of an acoustic biosensor

and signal processing, these innovations have paved the way for portable, scalable biosensor platforms suitable for point-of-care diagnostics and lab-on-a-chip devices.

2.4.1 History

The evolution of biosensor technology spans several decades, marked by gradual progress that culminated in rapid scientific and commercial breakthroughs. Although biosensors are now a cornerstone of modern analytical science, their history is relatively short. The foundational concept emerged in the mid-twentieth century and evolved slowly before gaining significant momentum in the 1970s and 1980s.

The origins of all biosensors, including piezoelectric biosensors, can be traced to the pioneering work of Professor Leland C. Clark Jr., often regarded as the father of the modern biosensor. In 1956, Clark published a seminal paper describing the oxygen electrode—a device that could quantitatively measure oxygen concentration using electrochemical principles. A few years later, in 1962, he introduced the idea of enhancing sensor intelligence by coupling enzymes to electrochemical transducers, thereby creating what he termed "enzyme electrodes." This innovation laid the groundwork for subsequent generations of biosensors that incorporated biological recognition elements such as enzymes, antibodies, and nucleic acids [60].

Despite this early innovation, biosensor development proceeded slowly for nearly 15 years. It was not until technological advances in microelectronics, materials science, and biochemistry converged that interest in the field began to accelerate. During the 1980s and 1990s, research activity expanded rapidly, leading to a wide range of biosensor designs tailored for clinical diagnostics, food safety testing, and environmental surveillance. This period also saw the emergence of commercial biosensor products, most notably glucose monitors for diabetic patients, which represented approximately 85% of the global biosensor market by the early 2000s. The scientific community's engagement with biosensor research has continued to grow exponentially. At the beginning of the millennium, around 950 publications addressed biosensor-related topics, a number that increased by nearly 60% in just 2 years and surpassed 2000 papers by 2005. The United States has consistently led in research output, followed by China, Japan, Germany, and the United Kingdom, countries that have all contributed substantially to the development of biosensor technologies and their integration into commercial and medical applications (Fig. 2.20).

Today, biosensors occupy a critical position in both academic and industrial research. What began as an experimental concept has evolved into a global industry valued at several billion dollars. The technological lineage of biosensors, from Clark's original enzyme electrode to sophisticated acoustic, optical, and electrochemical systems, reflects the dynamic interplay of interdisciplinary innovation [61]. This progression underscores how advances in physics, chemistry, biology, and engineering have collectively shaped the modern biosensor landscape.

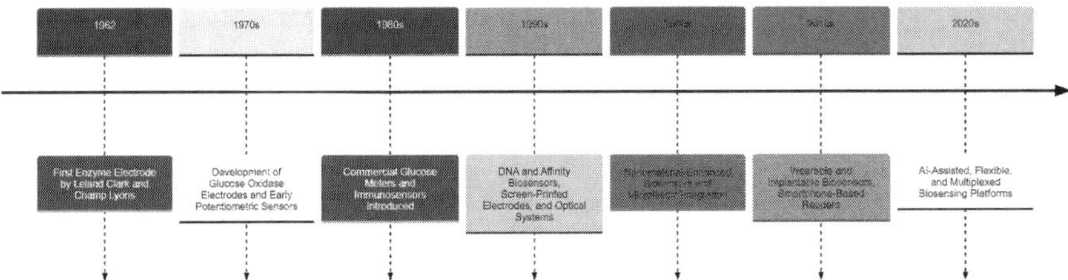

Fig. 2.20 Timeline of piezoelectric biosensors evolution

2.4.2 Types of Devices

The Quartz Crystal Microbalance Sensor

The **QCM** is a highly sensitive analytical instrument that measures minute mass variations on the order of nanograms to micrograms. Its precision and simplicity make it an indispensable tool for studying thin-film deposition, adsorption processes, and biomolecular interactions. The core of a QCM device is an AT-cut quartz crystal, which serves as a piezoelectric transducer oscillating at a specific resonant frequency. When material accumulates on its surface, the resonant frequency shifts in proportion to the added mass, enabling the quantification of nanoscale surface changes.

A typical QCM system comprises several integrated components that function together to generate, measure, and process oscillatory signals. The input circuitry connects the QCM sensor to the measurement system, conditioning the signal through amplification, filtering, and wave shaping. This ensures a stable digital signal for frequency analysis. A precise time base provides reference frequencies from crystal oscillators and counters, thereby establishing measurement accuracy. The control circuitry governs data acquisition and signal routing, while the counting and frequency-processing units measure the frequency output and convert it to digital data for display or computational analysis [62]. These subsystems collectively enable the QCM to detect mass variations with high temporal and frequency resolution.

The QCM operates on the inverse piezoelectric effect, in which an applied alternating voltage induces mechanical deformation in the quartz crystal. When an alternating current is applied across the crystal's electrodes, it oscillates in the thickness shear mode, vibrating parallel to its surface [63]. This mode of oscillation minimizes energy loss and ensures high-frequency stability, making it particularly suitable for measurements in liquid or gaseous environments.

Fundamental Frequency of Quartz

$$f_0 = \frac{n}{2t_q}\sqrt{\frac{\mu_q}{\rho_q}} \qquad (2.2)$$

This equation defines the *fundamental resonant frequency* (f_0) of a quartz crystal used in piezoelectric sensors, where:

- n = harmonic number (typically 1 for the fundamental mode)
- t_q = thickness of the quartz crystal
- μ_q = shear modulus of quartz
- ρ_q = density of quartz

The equation shows that the resonance frequency increases with stiffness (μ_q) and decreases with both density (ρ_q) and crystal thickness (t_q).

Sauerbrey Relation

$$\Delta f = -C \Delta m \tag{2.3}$$

This equation expresses the *frequency shift* (Δf) of a QCM as a result of a *mass change* (Δm) on its surface, where C is the Sauerbrey constant that depends on the crystal properties. The negative sign indicates that an increase in surface mass decreases the resonant frequency (Fig. 2.21).

Since its invention, the QCM has evolved significantly in both design and performance. The device's fundamental simplicity has facilitated its adaptation for numerous scientific and industrial applications. The fabrication process typically begins with preparing an AT-cut quartz crystal, which is oriented at approximately 35°25' relative to the z-axis to ensure optimal piezoelectric performance. The crystal's thickness determines its operating frequency; thinner crystals have higher resonant frequencies.

Fabrication involves several key steps. The quartz substrate is first cleaned to remove organic contaminants, ensuring a pristine surface for subsequent processing. Photolithography is then used to define the electrode pattern: a photoresist layer is applied, exposed through a photomask, and developed to create the desired geometry. Following this, a thin adhesion layer, commonly chromium or titanium—is deposited, followed by the electrode material, typically gold or platinum [64]. The lift-off process removes excess photoresist, leaving behind the electrode pattern. The same procedure is repeated on the opposite side of the crystal to form the bottom electrode. Gold and platinum are preferred due to their high conductivity, chemical stability, and inertness. In recent years, micromachining and lithographic techniques have enabled the production of multichannel QCM arrays on a single quartz substrate. These arrays allow simultaneous measurement of multiple analytes or reference samples, improving throughput and reducing experimental variability. Advanced QCM structures, such as MESA (Micro-Electro-Systems Arrays), have been developed to minimize acoustic interference between channels, ensuring that each resonator operates independently with minimal cross-talk.

Surface Acoustic Wave (SAW) Sensors
SAW sensors represent a class of piezoelectric devices that utilize the propagation of acoustic waves along the surface of a solid substrate to detect physical, chemical, or biological changes in their environment. Since their conceptual introduction in

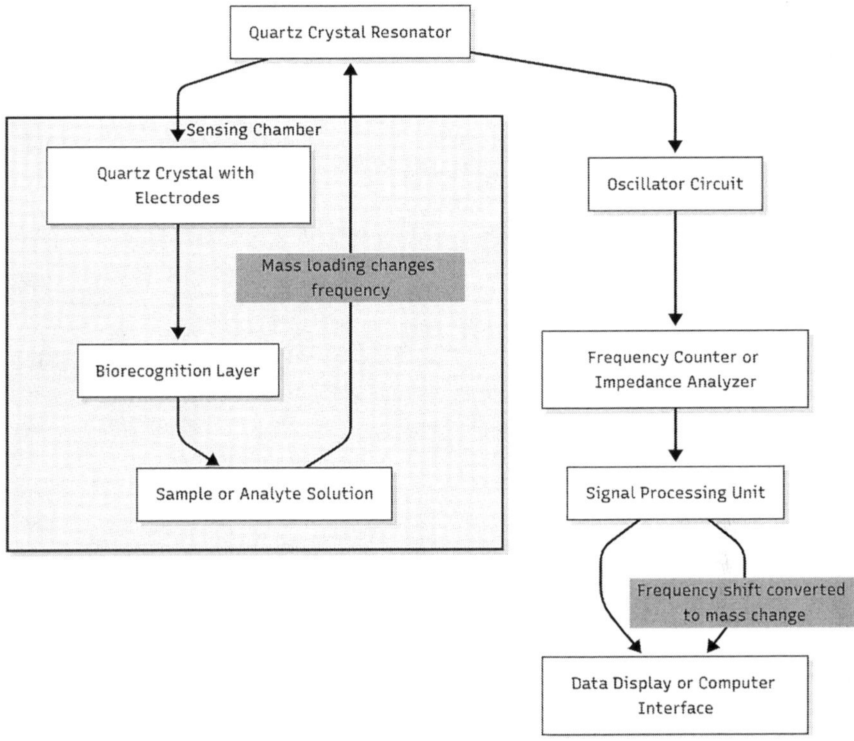

Fig. 2.21 QCM system architecture

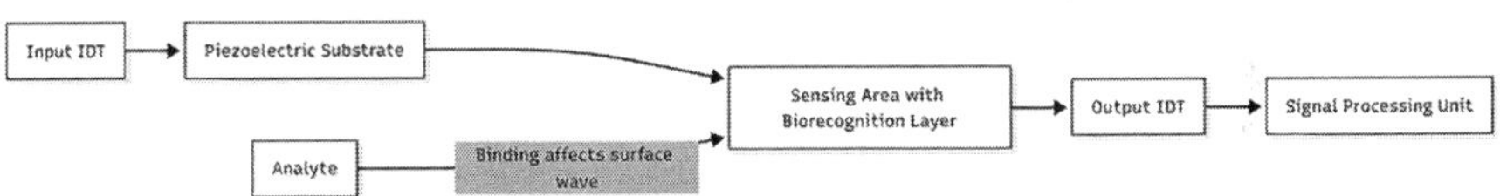

Fig. 2.22 SAW device layout

the 1960s, SAW sensors have evolved into highly versatile and precise tools for monitoring parameters such as pressure, temperature, humidity, and gas composition [65]. Their compact design, passive operation, and compatibility with integrated circuits make them especially well-suited for modern applications in environmental sensing, industrial monitoring, and biomedical diagnostics (Fig. 2.22).

The development of SAW sensors began in the mid-1960s when researchers first proposed the concept of surface acoustic wave propagation on piezoelectric substrates. During the 1970s, these devices found early commercial applications in radar and television systems, primarily serving as filters for high-frequency signal processing. The 1980s marked a turning point as SAW devices were adapted for gas sensing, exploiting their ability to detect mass and viscoelastic changes on the substrate surface. By the 1990s, researchers had extended SAW technology into biosensing, enabling the detection of biological molecules and humidity variations through selective surface coatings.

In the early 2000s, the emergence of wireless, passive SAW sensors enabled their use in harsh or inaccessible environments, where they could operate without internal power sources. The 2010s brought further advances through the integration of microfluidics, nanomaterials, and flexible substrates, improving sensitivity and miniaturization. Over the past decade, SAW sensors have been refined for advanced biomedical and diagnostic applications, including COVID-19 detection, aptamer-based assays, and graphene-enhanced sensing, solidifying their role as cutting-edge biosensing platforms.

A SAW sensor typically consists of a piezoelectric substrate, a set of interdigital transducers (IDTs), and reflective elements that shape and direct the acoustic wave. The IDTs, fine metallic electrodes patterned on the substrate, serve as both transmitters and receivers of acoustic waves [66]. When an alternating electrical signal is applied to the input IDT, it generates a mechanical surface wave through the piezoelectric effect. This wave travels across the substrate's surface and is either absorbed, reflected, or modulated by changes in surface properties. The output IDT then converts the returning or modified acoustic wave back into an electrical signal, completing the transduction process.

Two main SAW sensor configurations are commonly used: delay line and resonator types. In delay-line devices, the acoustic wave propagates freely between the transmitting and receiving IDTs, enabling precise measurement of time-dependent or phase-shifted signals. Resonator-type SAW sensors, on the other hand, confine acoustic energy between two reflective gratings, forming a standing-wave cavity. This structure enhances signal amplitude and improves measurement resolution, making resonator designs particularly useful for high-sensitivity applications.

The performance of a SAW device depends heavily on the substrate material and the IDT design. Quartz, lithium niobate, and lithium tantalate are frequently used substrates due to their strong piezoelectric response and mechanical stability. The wave velocity and frequency, typically in the range of tens of megahertz to several gigahertz, are influenced by factors such as electrode spacing, crystal orientation, and surface coatings.

SAW sensors operate on the fundamental principle that any interaction at the sensor's surface alters the propagation characteristics of the acoustic wave. These interactions can include mass loading, changes in elasticity, variations in temperature, or adsorption of target analytes. Such modifications result in measurable shifts in wave velocity, amplitude, or phase, which are subsequently translated into corresponding changes in electrical output [67].

In biosensing applications, the surface of the piezoelectric substrate is functionalized with a biological recognition element, such as an antibody, enzyme, or DNA probe, that selectively binds to the target analyte. The binding event increases the effective surface mass or alters the viscoelastic properties of the sensing layer, resulting in a detectable frequency shift. Because acoustic waves are confined near the surface (typically within a few wavelengths of depth), SAW sensors exhibit exceptional sensitivity to surface-level changes, enabling the detection of minute amounts of biological material.

Wireless passive SAW sensors have gained significant attention for remote monitoring applications. These systems typically include a transceiver, a SAW device, and an antenna. The transceiver sends an interrogation signal, which the SAW device converts into an acoustic wave. The modified wave is then reflected back to the transceiver, carrying encoded information about the measured parameter. This configuration enables fully passive operation, requiring no internal power source, and allows data transmission over long distances with high precision and stability.

SAW sensors have demonstrated broad applicability across multiple fields. In industrial and power systems, they are used to monitor temperature, pressure, and strain in components subjected to high voltage and mechanical stress. Their wireless operation and robustness make them ideal for use in smart substations and energy infrastructure, where continuous monitoring is necessary without direct electrical contact [68]. In the transportation sector, SAW sensors have been integrated into train axles to monitor friction-induced temperature changes and detect early signs of mechanical wear, preventing failures and ensuring safety.

In environmental science, SAW sensors are widely employed for humidity and gas detection. Their selective coatings enable the adsorption of specific gases or water vapor, producing measurable frequency shifts proportional to their concentrations. This makes them valuable for applications ranging from air quality monitoring to industrial process control.

More recently, SAW sensors have emerged as promising candidates in biomedical diagnostics. Functionalized with biorecognition layers, they can detect biomarkers, pathogens, and genetic material with high sensitivity and specificity. Their ability to operate label-free and in real time provides distinct advantages for clinical testing, such as rapid infection detection and continuous health monitoring.

2.4.3 Technical Characteristics

A biosensor is a hybrid analytical device that integrates biological recognition elements with a physicochemical transducer to convert a biological interaction into a measurable signal. The essential components of a biosensor include a bioreceptor, a transducer, and a signal processing system. Together, these components enable the selective detection, conversion, and quantification of analytes in complex samples.

The bioreceptor serves as the sensing interface that specifically recognizes the target molecule or organism. Depending on the application, this component can consist of enzymes, antibodies, nucleic acids, aptamers, or synthetic recognition materials such as molecularly imprinted polymers. The interaction between the bioreceptor and analyte generates a physicochemical change—such as mass addition, heat release, charge transfer, or refractive index variation—that is then detected by the transducer.

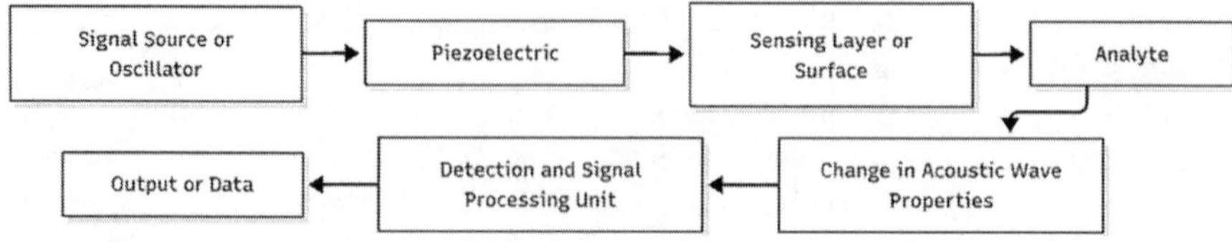

Fig. 2.23 Functional blocks of an acoustic biosensor system

The transducer converts this biological event into an electrical signal. Its type determines the biosensor's operational principle, electrochemical, optical, acoustic, or piezoelectric. In the case of QCM and SAW biosensors, the transduction is based on the piezoelectric effect. When a biological interaction occurs at the sensor surface, the additional mass or alteration in the viscoelastic properties of the piezoelectric material changes its oscillation frequency or wave velocity [69]. These frequency shifts are directly proportional to the amount of analyte bound to the surface, allowing quantitative measurement (Fig. 2.23).

For QCM biosensors, the quartz crystal acts as the core sensing element. The alternating electrical signal applied to the crystal induces oscillations at its resonant frequency. When biomolecules bind to the crystal surface, the added mass causes a measurable decrease in frequency. The output signal is conditioned by a microbalance preprocessor, converted into a digital waveform, and analyzed using a frequency counter or computer interface. This configuration enables real-time monitoring of binding kinetics without the need for fluorescent or radioactive labeling.

SAW biosensors function similarly but rely on acoustic waves that propagate along the surface of a piezoelectric substrate. The surface is functionalized with a bioreceptor layer that captures the target analyte. The interaction modifies the acoustic wave's velocity or amplitude, which is then translated into an electrical signal by interdigital transducers. This label-free, surface-sensitive mechanism allows SAW sensors to achieve rapid response times and high detection sensitivity, even for low analyte concentrations.

2.4.4   Clinical Applications

The use of acoustic biosensors, particularly QCM systems, in pathogen detection and molecular diagnostics has expanded rapidly due to their exceptional sensitivity and ability to operate without labeling agents. These sensors can identify infectious agents, nucleic acids, and proteins associated with disease within short assay times, often matching or surpassing the performance of traditional diagnostic methods.

Extensive research has focused on the application of QCM-based immunosensors and aptasensors for detecting viral and bacterial pathogens. For instance, in influenza virus detection, QCM immunosensors have achieved detection ranges of

10^3–10^7 PFU/mL, which closely match viral titers observed in nasal wash samples from infected individuals. When nanobead amplification was incorporated, the detection limit improved by two orders of magnitude, enabling accurate measurement of viral concentrations even in dilute samples. Similarly, nanowell-based aptasensors have achieved rapid detection within 10 min, comparable to the time required for commercial rapid diagnostic tests (RDTs), while maintaining quantitative precision.

In hepatitis B virus (HBV) diagnostics, a QCM system employing rolling circle amplification (RCA) demonstrated highly effective performance. The RCA-QCM device completed both amplification and detection within an hour, eliminating the need for thermal cyclers typically required in PCR assays. When tested on HBV-positive clinical samples, the RCA-QCM showed 96% correlation with real-time PCR results, highlighting its potential as a cost-effective, portable diagnostic tool.

QCM-based biosensors have also proven effective in detecting parasitic and bacterial infections, offering greater sensitivity and accuracy than microscopy and other conventional tests such as dot-blot assays or shell vial cultures. For example, QCM immunosensors achieved detection limits as low as 2 ng/mL—comparable to those of ELISA—across a wide dynamic range spanning several orders of magnitude [70]. In assays designed to measure multiple biomarkers simultaneously, these systems have achieved detection limits in the femtogram per milliliter (fg/mL) range, enabling ultra-sensitive quantification of trace biomolecules in mixed samples.

One of the major technological advancements in this area is the wireless-electrode Quartz Crystal Microbalance (WE-QCM). Unlike traditional QCM sensors that rely on metallic electrode coatings, the WE-QCM uses a bare quartz surface, which eliminates electrode degradation during cleaning or chemical regeneration. Because the quartz surface itself is chemically stable and resistant to acid or alkali treatment, it can be reused indefinitely, making the system replacement-free and cost-efficient. Moreover, the bare quartz surface of a WE-QCM exhibits strong affinity for protein adsorption, allowing receptor molecules to be immobilized directly without the use of linkers or self-assembled monolayers. This direct immobilization significantly simplifies biosensor fabrication. Streptavidin, for instance, binds strongly to the quartz surface and can serve as a base layer for capturing biotin-conjugated receptors. Since inactive proteins such as bovine serum albumin (BSA) can block remaining surface sites, the sensor surface can be reused multiple times without loss of activity, further reducing operational costs. The high sensitivity of WE-QCM technology enables detailed studies of the binding affinity between biomolecules. By analyzing the frequency changes over time, researchers can assess how the affinity constant varies with analyte concentration. This is particularly useful for characterizing complex interactions, such as those between immunoglobulin G (IgG) and protein A, which exhibit concentration-dependent structural variations. In binding experiments, the exponential decrease in oscillation frequency reflects the rate and strength of molecular association. At higher analyte concentrations, steric hindrance and spatial crowding on the sensor surface can reduce binding efficiency by blocking active sites [71]. However, the extreme sensitivity of WE-QCM enables the accurate characterization of these kinetic effects, allowing the precise determination of equilibrium and rate constants for biomolecular interactions (Table 2.15).

Table 2.15 Representative pathogen detection studies using QCM

Target	Sensor type	Recognition element	Detection limit	Assay time
Influenza virus	QCM immunosensor	Antibody	10^3 PFU/mL	<10 min
HBV	RCA-QCM	DNA probe	pg/mL	$\approx$1 h
E. coli	QCM immunosensor	Antibody	2 ng/mL	20 min
Salmonella	SAW biosensor	Aptamer	10^2 CFU/mL	30 min

Taken together, QCM and WE-QCM systems combine high sensitivity, quantitative accuracy, and reusability, making them strong candidates for next-generation molecular diagnostic platforms. Their rapid response, compatibility with microfluidic systems, and potential for miniaturization align well with the global trend toward point-of-care testing—a shift that emphasizes portable, fast, and reliable tools for early disease detection and continuous patient monitoring.

2.4.5 Regulatory Considerations

For immunosensors to transition from laboratory research to clinical use, they must meet strict regulatory requirements that ensure their safety, reliability, and performance. These requirements involve multiple stages, analytical validation, clinical validation, and formal approval from relevant regulatory authorities. The goal is to confirm that the device produces consistent, accurate results suitable for medical diagnostics. Within the European Union, biosensors intended for diagnostic use fall under the In Vitro Diagnostic Medical Devices Regulation (IVDR). This framework governs the manufacturing, testing, and commercialization of diagnostic devices, including immunosensors. Products that meet IVDR standards receive CE marking, which indicates compliance with essential safety, performance, and quality requirements [72]. The CE mark allows the product to be sold throughout EU member states and in many countries that recognize EU conformity standards. The CE marking process requires the manufacturer to demonstrate that the biosensor performs as intended, poses no risks to users or patients, and meets applicable quality management standards. Depending on the device's classification and risk level, this process may involve internal testing, third-party audits, and performance evaluations based on published data or clinical studies. Once approved, the manufacturer must maintain ongoing quality assurance and participate in periodic audits to ensure continued compliance.

In the United States, immunosensors and other diagnostic devices are regulated by the FDA. To enter the market, a biosensor must either obtain premarket approval (PMA) or receive clearance through the 510(k) process, which demonstrates that the new device is substantially equivalent to an existing, legally marketed product. Unlike the CE mark, FDA approval generally requires comprehensive clinical trials that directly assess the device's safety and efficacy in patient populations.

Although both systems share the same fundamental purpose, ensuring the safety and effectiveness of new medical devices, they differ in procedure and scope. FDA approval tends to be more stringent and limited to the U.S. market. In contrast, CE marking is internationally recognized and facilitates faster access to the European and global markets. Because the CE process relies partly on clinical evaluations and literature reviews of equivalent devices, it allows new technologies to reach patients more quickly, especially those addressing unmet clinical needs.

The European model places greater responsibility on manufacturers, requiring them to implement robust post-market surveillance and quality control systems to monitor device performance. Companies undergo regular audits and are required to document adverse events or product modifications [73]. In this framework, clinical safety and effectiveness are assessed not only during pre-market testing but also continuously throughout the device's lifecycle (Fig. 2.24).

By comparison, FDA-regulated devices must complete rigorous, large-scale clinical trials before approval. These trials are often viewed as gold-standard studies, generating high-quality data that advance scientific understanding and establish strong evidence of clinical value. Once approved, a device must adhere to the FDA's Good Manufacturing Practice (GMP) and Quality System Regulation (QSR) standards to maintain its approval status.

2.5   Electrical and Field-Effect Biosensors

Biosensors are analytical devices designed to detect and measure the presence or concentration of biological substances. These substances, or analytes, can include biomolecules, cells, microorganisms, or larger biological structures. A typical biosensor comprises four essential components: the analyte being investigated, a biorecognition element that specifically binds to the analyte, a transducer that converts the biological interaction into a measurable signal, and a processor that interprets the signal into a meaningful output (Fig. 2.25).

The earliest biosensor was introduced by Clark and Lyons in 1962 to measure glucose levels. This device used the enzyme glucose oxidase, which catalyzed the conversion of glucose into gluconic acid. The reaction caused a measurable change in pH, allowing glucose concentration to be determined from the corresponding shift in acidity. Since that pioneering work, biosensors have evolved into highly versatile tools capable of detecting a wide range of analytes, from small molecules such as glucose and urea to macromolecules like DNA, antigens, and antibodies [74]. In modern applications, they can even be used for real-time monitoring of cells, tissues, and physiological parameters within living systems.

Today, biosensors play a vital role in healthcare diagnostics, environmental testing, food quality control, and biotechnology. Depending on the specific analyte and detection principle, biosensors can be designed to measure various physical or chemical signals, most commonly electrical, optical, or mechanical. In clinical settings, they are invaluable for monitoring disease biomarkers, with glucose

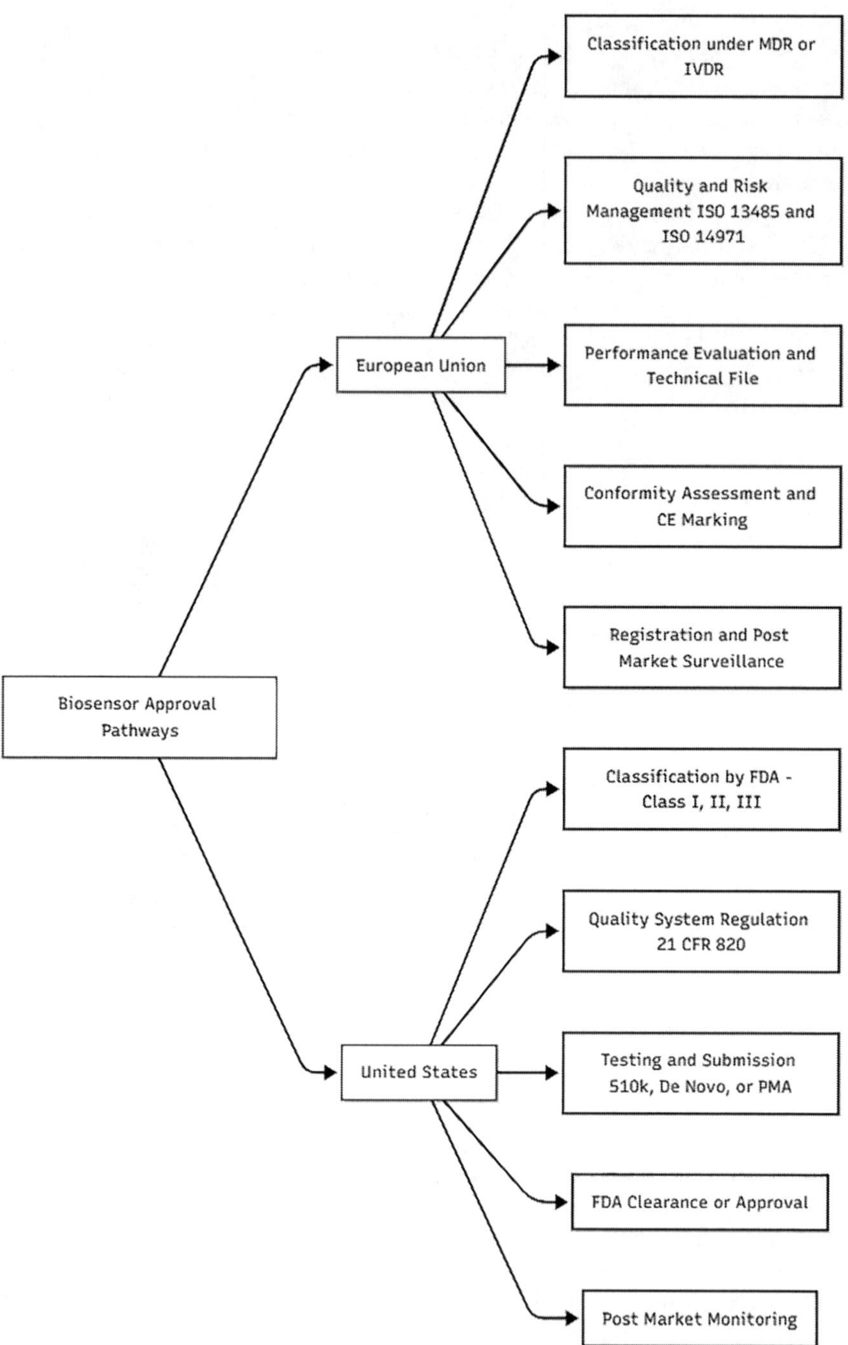

Fig. 2.24 Approval pathways for biosensors (EU vs. US)

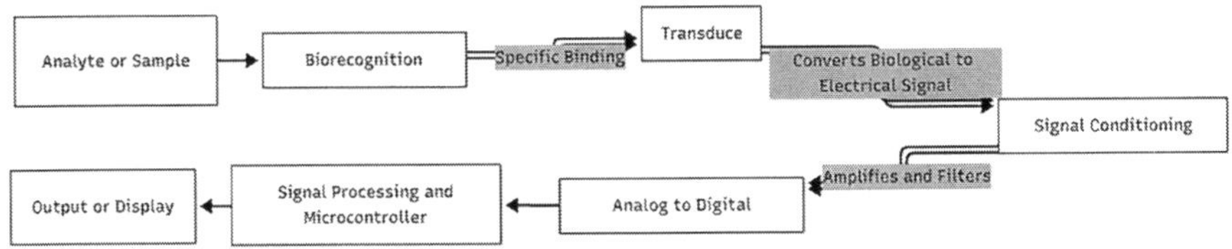

Fig. 2.25 Structure of a typical electrical biosensor

monitoring in diabetes management among the most recognized examples. The ability of biosensors to provide rapid, reliable, and quantitative data continues to make them indispensable in both laboratory and point-of-care settings.

2.5.1 History

The foundation of FET technology, which later gave rise to FET-based biosensors, dates back to the early twentieth century. Researchers such as Julius Edgar Lilienfeld and Oskar Heil were among the first to propose devices capable of controlling current flow using an electric field, though the available technology at the time could not realize these designs. The modern transistor era began in 1947 at Bell Laboratories, where William Shockley, John Bardeen, and Walter Brattain developed the first working transistor, paving the way for subsequent advances in semiconductor physics.

In the 1950s and 1960s, further breakthroughs at Bell Labs led to the development of the metal–oxide–semiconductor field-effect transistor (MOSFET), made possible through the discovery of silicon dioxide surface passivation. This progress enabled the miniaturization and planar construction of transistors, an essential step toward integrated circuits and, eventually, biosensor technology. Around the same time, in 1962, Leland C. Clark and Champ Lyons introduced the first enzyme-based biosensor, demonstrating how biochemical reactions could be integrated with electronic detection systems.

By 1970, Piet Bergveld developed the first ion-sensitive field-effect transistor (ISFET), marking the beginning of the BioFET family of sensors [75]. Unlike conventional MOSFETs, the ISFET replaced the metal gate with an ion-sensitive membrane, an electrolyte solution, and a reference electrode, allowing it to directly detect changes in ion concentration. Subsequent innovations followed rapidly, including the adsorption FET (ADFET), patented by P. F. Cox in 1974, and the hydrogen-sensitive MOSFET, demonstrated by I. Lundstrom and colleagues in 1975.

Through the 1980s and 1990s, a variety of specialized BioFETs emerged: the gas-sensitive FET (GASFET), pressure-sensitive FET (PRESSFET), enzyme-modified FET (ENFET), immunologically modified FET (IMFET), and DNA-specific FET (DNAFET). These devices expanded the capabilities of FET biosensors into diverse biomedical and environmental applications. By the early 2000s, advancements such as gene-modified FETs (GenFETs) and cell-potential FETs (CPFETs) had been developed, followed more recently by organic electrolyte-gated FETs (OEGFETs), which combine flexibility, low operating voltage, and enhanced biocompatibility (Fig. 2.26).

Collectively, these innovations have transformed FET-based biosensors into powerful tools capable of measuring a wide array of physical, chemical, and biological parameters. They remain at the forefront of modern diagnostic technologies due to their rapid response, scalability, and compatibility with microelectronics and nanomaterials.

2.5.2 Technical Characteristics

Hardware

A FET biosensor is composed of two fundamental components: the biorecognition section and the signal transduction section. The biorecognition section serves as the interface between the sensor and the biological sample. It contains a buffer medium that maintains physiological conditions, biorecognition probes that selectively bind to the target analyte, and linkers that immobilize these probes on the sensor surface. Common buffers, such as phosphate-buffered saline, Tris-buffered saline, or sodium citrate, are used to sustain biomolecular structure and function [76]. These buffers not only provide a stable environment for molecular interactions but also act as gate electrolytes, establishing electrical contact between the gate electrode and the transistor channel.

The biorecognition probes can be natural biological elements, such as antibodies, cell membranes, or CRISPR/Cas complexes, or synthetic entities, such as aptamers, peptides, and small organic molecules. Their high binding specificity allows the biosensor to identify and quantify target molecules even within complex biological fluids. Probes are typically attached to the channel surface either physically, through non-covalent interactions such as hydrogen bonding or electrostatic attraction, or chemically, through covalent bonding that enhances long-term stability.

The signal transduction section relies on a high-performance transistor that converts biological recognition events into measurable electrical signals. Structurally, the device comprises three electrodes, source, drain, and gate, connected through a semiconducting channel positioned on an insulating substrate. Gold is the most

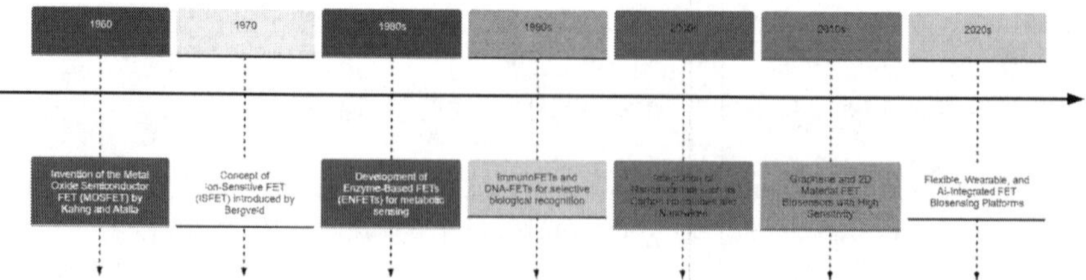

Fig. 2.26 Timeline of FET biosensor history

commonly used electrode material because of its conductivity and chemical inertness, although intermediate adhesion layers of chromium, titanium, or nickel are often added to strengthen the bond between the metal and the substrate.

The semiconductor channel acts as the active region where electrical conduction occurs and where sensing events are detected. In n-type channels, electrons are the primary charge carriers and conduct current when a positive gate voltage is applied, whereas in p-type channels, holes serve this function under a negative gate bias. The gate voltage controls the charge distribution in the channel via the dielectric layer, typically silicon dioxide, aluminum oxide, or hafnium oxide, modulating current between the source and drain electrodes [77].

Modern FET biosensors often employ liquid-gate configurations, in which the gate voltage is applied directly through the electrolyte using a silver/silver chloride electrode. This setup allows the device to operate at low voltages, usually below 1 volt, improving sensitivity and reducing energy consumption. The liquid-gated configuration also enhances signal-to-noise performance, enabling real-time monitoring of biochemical reactions under near-physiological conditions (Table 2.16).

The sensing mechanism of an FET biosensor is based on the modulation of electrical charge near the channel surface in response to biochemical interactions. When a gate voltage is applied, the device behaves as a capacitor, with the gate and channel serving as the two plates separated by the dielectric. Any change in charge distribution, caused by biomolecular binding, variations in ion concentration, or enzymatic activity, alters the potential difference across the gate and channel.

This shift in potential alters the carrier density and mobility in the semiconductor channel, leading to measurable variations in current between the source and drain [78]. Essentially, the biosensor translates the electrostatic or charge-transfer effects of molecular recognition into electrical signals that can be amplified and recorded. Positively or negatively charged analytes influence the local electric field, changing the threshold voltage and drain current. In this way, the sensor provides a direct electrical readout of biological events, such as DNA hybridization, antigen–antibody binding, or enzymatic reactions.

$$\Delta V_T = \frac{Q_b}{C_{ox}} \tag{2.4}$$

where Q_b = surface charge resulting from binding, and C_{ox} = oxide capacitance per unit area.

Table 2.16 Typical materials used in BioFET construction

Component	Common materials	Desired properties
Substrate	Si, glass, polymer	Mechanical stability
Electrodes	Au (+ Cr/Ti adhesion)	Conductive/inert
Dielectric	SiO_2, Al_2O_3, HfO_2	High κ insulation
Channel	Si, graphene, CNTs, MoS_2	High mobility, biocompatible
Biolayer	Enzyme, antibody, DNA, aptamer	Selective binding

This equation describes how the threshold voltage (ΔV_T) in field-effect biosensors shifts due to charge accumulation at the sensing surface. A higher surface charge or lower oxide capacitance increases the voltage shift, thereby influencing the device's transduction efficiency and sensitivity.

Software

The software integrated into FET biosensor systems plays a pivotal role in data processing, analysis, and visualization. When biological interactions occur on the sensor surface, they generate changes in voltage or current that must be accurately captured and interpreted. The software filters noise and corrects for signal fluctuations caused by environmental factors, ensuring that the data reflect true biomolecular activity rather than artifacts. Digital signal processing algorithms convert the analog electrical output into numerical values, which are then analyzed using computational models. Advanced software packages often incorporate mathematical fitting and equivalent circuit modeling to interpret the relationship between charge transfer and analyte concentration [79]. Increasingly, AI and machine learning algorithms are being implemented to recognize signal patterns, detect anomalies, and improve the predictive accuracy of biosensor data. The software also handles automatic calibration, compensating for drift or sensor degradation over time. It can visualize results through intuitive interfaces that display graphs, concentration curves, or color-coded indicators, allowing researchers and clinicians to quickly assess the sample's characteristics. Additionally, wireless connectivity features such as Bluetooth or Wi-Fi enable data transmission to external devices, laboratory servers, or cloud-based databases for storage and further analysis (Table 2.17).

In modern medical and laboratory applications, the integration of intelligent software transforms FET biosensors from simple electrical devices into smart analytical systems. These systems not only detect molecular interactions with precision but also interpret and communicate findings in real time, supporting rapid diagnostics and continuous health monitoring.

2.5.3 Types of Devices

Electrical biosensors occupy a leading position in analytical and biomedical technologies due to their exceptional sensitivity, rapid response, and ability to be miniaturized for portable, real-time applications. They function by using a biological

Table 2.17 Core software functions

Function	Description	Benefit
Filtering	Removes drift/environmental noise	Stable baseline
Calibration	Auto-adjusts reference levels	Accuracy
Modeling	Equivalent-circuit or AI fitting	Quantitative analysis
Visualization	Graphs & dashboards	User-friendly output
Connectivity	Bluetooth/Wi-Fi/Cloud	Remote monitoring

recognition element to selectively bind to a target analyte. This biological interaction is then translated into an electrical signal through a transducer, which can measure changes in current, voltage, conductivity, or impedance. The resulting data can be analyzed quantitatively, making these biosensors indispensable for clinical diagnostics, environmental monitoring, and biotechnological research.

The significance of electrical biosensors lies in their ability to convert biological recognition events into precise electrical outputs. This characteristic enables their use in numerous applications, including glucose monitoring in diabetes, pathogen detection, toxic compound identification, and environmental pollutant tracking [80]. As a result, they serve as the technological bridge between biochemical systems and electronic readout platforms, supporting the ongoing shift from traditional laboratory-based testing to portable, automated, and point-of-care diagnostic systems. Electrical biosensors can be categorized by the electrical parameter they measure. The main classifications include electrochemical, capacitive, impedimetric, and FET-based biosensors, as well as hybrid designs that integrate multiple detection principles (Table 2.18).

FET-based biosensors, or **BioFETs**, represent a distinct class of devices that detect target molecules by modulating semiconductor conductivity. In these devices, biological interactions at the sensor surface alter the local electric field, thereby altering the current flowing through the transistor channel. Different variants exist, such as the ion-sensitive FET (ISFET), enzyme-modified FET (ENFET), and DNA-FET, each tailored to specific analytes and biological recognition mechanisms.

FET-based biosensors can be classified according to the type of bioreceptor immobilized on the transistor surface and the nature of the analyte being detected. Each variant is designed to recognize specific biological or chemical species through different transduction mechanisms. The fundamental distinctions among these biosensors lie in their recognition mechanism, whether enzymatic catalysis, molecular binding, or cellular activity, and in the type of signal they generate upon target interaction.

The earliest and most established FET biosensor is the **ISFET.** Unlike a traditional transistor, the ISFET replaces the metal gate with an ion-sensitive membrane and an electrolyte solution connected to a reference electrode. When exposed to an analyte, changes in ion concentration, most notably hydrogen ions, alter the

Table 2.18 Characteristic parameters of electrical biosensor types

Type	Measured variable	Typical transducer	Sensitivity	Example application
Amperometric	Current	Enzyme electrode	High	Glucose testing
Potentiometric	Potential	ISFET	Moderate	pH monitoring
Conductometric	Conductivity	Planar electrodes	Medium	Urea assays
Capacitive	Capacitance	Metal–insulator–metal	Very high	Protein binding
Impedimetric	Impedance	Microelectrode array	High	Cell analysis
Field effect	Channel current	BioFET	Very high	DNA or antigen sensing

membrane's surface potential, thereby altering channel conductivity [81]. Because of this sensitivity to ionic variations, ISFETs are widely used for pH measurement, monitoring enzymatic reactions, and studying ion dynamics in biological fluids.

Another important variant is the **Enzyme Field-Effect Transistor (EnFET),** which builds upon the ISFET design by adding a layer of immobilized enzymes. These enzymes catalyze specific biochemical reactions that produce or consume charged species, such as protons, thereby causing measurable electrical changes in the transistor's output. EnFETs are particularly valuable in medical diagnostics and biotechnology, where they are used to monitor metabolites such as glucose, urea, or lactate in blood and tissue samples.

The **Immuno Field-Effect Transistor (ImmunoFET)** utilizes antibodies as biorecognition elements. When a specific antigen binds to the immobilized antibody on the transistor surface, the local charge distribution changes, resulting in a detectable shift in the channel current. This mechanism enables ImmunoFETs to identify pathogens, disease biomarkers, and other antigenic molecules with high specificity. Such sensors have been developed to detect infectious agents, such as bacteria and viruses, as well as protein markers associated with cancer and cardiovascular disease.

A related category, the **DNA Field-Effect Transistor (DNA-FET),** also known as a genosensor, employs single-stranded DNA or RNA probes that hybridize to complementary nucleic acid sequences. Hybridization alters the surface charge density, causing measurable variations in current or voltage across the transistor. DNA-FETs are widely used in genetic analysis, pathogen detection, and mutation screening, offering rapid, label-free alternatives to conventional molecular diagnostic methods.

In more complex systems, **Cell-Based FETs** (Cellular BioFETs) integrate living cells as sensing elements. These devices monitor cellular responses such as changes in membrane potential, ion exchange, or metabolite secretion. The biological activity of the immobilized cells directly modulates the transistor's electrical characteristics, enabling real-time observation of cell viability, toxic effects, and pharmacological responses. Such biosensors hold significant promise in drug discovery, toxicology, and physiological research.

Beyond these core types, **hybrid and multifunctional BioFETs** are being developed to combine multiple sensing mechanisms within a single platform. For example, an EnFET can be integrated with an ISFET to measure both pH and metabolic by-products simultaneously. Similarly, nanomaterial-based transistors—such as graphene or carbon nanotube FETs—are enhancing sensitivity and expanding detection capabilities to ultra-low concentrations (Fig. 2.27).

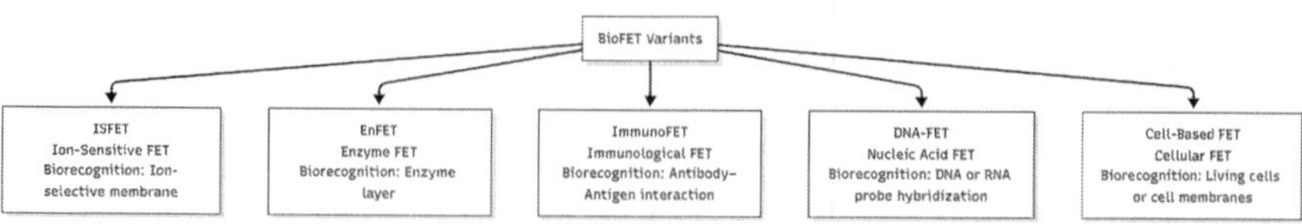

Fig. 2.27 Variants of BioFETs

The diversity of FET biosensors underscores their adaptability to a broad range of analytical challenges. From detecting single ions to monitoring entire cellular processes, these devices exemplify the convergence of microelectronics, surface chemistry, and molecular biology. Their continuous evolution reflects the growing demand for precise, fast, and miniaturized diagnostic technologies in medicine, biotechnology, and environmental science.

2.5.4   Clinical Applications

BioFETs, have emerged as powerful analytical tools for detecting biomolecules in real time. Their ability to detect electrical charge variations near the sensor surface makes them exceptionally sensitive and selective, enabling rapid identification of target molecules, including proteins, nucleic acids, hormones, and disease biomarkers [82]. Because BioFETs provide label-free and instantaneous electrical readouts, they are well-suited for modern medical diagnostics that demand speed, precision, and miniaturization.

BioFET sensors have demonstrated great potential in the rapid detection of infectious diseases. During the COVID-19 pandemic, BioFETs functionalized with antibodies specific to the SARS-CoV-2 spike protein enabled direct viral detection from nasal swab samples within minutes, without requiring amplification or labeling. These sensors offered an affordable and fast alternative to polymerase chain reaction (PCR) assays. Beyond SARS-CoV-2, similar devices have been developed to detect pathogens such as HIV, hepatitis B and C, Zika virus, and influenza. Their short analysis time, minimal sample preparation, and compatibility with portable formats make them highly valuable for large-scale screening and field diagnostics.

In oncology, BioFET sensors play an essential role in detecting circulating tumor biomarkers in blood and other biological fluids. For instance, prostate-specific antigen (PSA) detection enables early diagnosis of prostate cancer, while HER2 receptor sensing supports breast cancer monitoring and treatment selection. These devices can measure biomarkers at extremely low concentrations, often in the femtomolar range, enabling non-invasive, real-time evaluation of disease progression or therapeutic response. Their compact size and electronic readout allow integration into point-of-care diagnostic tools for routine use in clinics and personalized medicine.

Enzyme-modified FETs (EnFETs) functionalized with glucose oxidase are among the most widely applied BioFET systems in clinical medicine. These sensors continuously monitor glucose concentrations in blood, sweat, or interstitial fluid by measuring the ionic changes generated during the enzymatic oxidation of glucose. The main advantage lies in the possibility of non-invasive or minimally invasive detection through wearable technologies such as smart patches, contact lenses, or wristbands [83]. Compared to conventional glucometers, FET-based glucose sensors offer continuous monitoring and improved comfort for patients requiring long-term glycemic control.

BioFET sensors are increasingly used in **endocrinology** to quantify hormones such as cortisol, insulin, and thyroid hormones. Cortisol testing helps diagnose stress-related and adrenal disorders, while insulin and thyroid hormone measurements are valuable for managing diabetes and thyroid dysfunction. These biosensors provide rapid, precise hormonal profiling, enabling personalized treatment adjustments and continuous physiological monitoring beyond traditional laboratory settings.

In **neuroscience**, BioFETs enable the detection of neurotransmitters and disease-related biomarkers. Devices designed to measure dopamine and serotonin levels are used to assess mood disorders and monitor Parkinson's disease. Similarly, sensors targeting β-amyloid and tau proteins have been developed for early diagnosis of Alzheimer's disease. The real-time electrical output of BioFETs provides immediate feedback on neurochemical fluctuations, facilitating both research and clinical applications in brain health monitoring.

The miniaturized nature of BioFETs allows their integration into wearable and implantable devices for continuous health monitoring. These systems form the foundation of personalized medicine by enabling real-time tracking of individual biochemical markers and treatment responses. Combined with lab-on-a-chip technologies, FET biosensors can simultaneously analyze multiple biomarkers from very small sample volumes, offering fast, cost-effective, and automated diagnostics at the patient's bedside. Such integration reduces reliance on centralized laboratories and expands access to precision healthcare, especially in remote or resource-limited environments.

2.5.5 *Regulatory Considerations*

Before FET biosensors, particularly implantable or wearable devices, can be introduced into clinical use, it is essential to address both ethical and regulatory considerations. These aspects ensure patient safety, data protection, and compliance with medical device standards throughout the product's lifecycle, from design and testing to manufacturing and post-market surveillance. From an ethical standpoint, the use of FET-based biosensors in healthcare requires fully informed patient consent [84]. Individuals must clearly understand the benefits, risks, and possible implications of using these devices. This includes the potential for continuous health monitoring, data collection, and integration with digital health platforms. Transparency about how personal health data will be collected, stored, used, and shared is vital. Robust privacy safeguards must be established to prevent unauthorized access or misuse of patient information.

Regulatory compliance begins with rigorous biocompatibility and safety testing. Any biosensor intended for long-term or implantable use must undergo extensive preclinical and clinical evaluations to verify its safety, reliability, and stability within biological environments. These tests assess not only the device's functionality but also potential side effects, toxicity, and compatibility with tissues and body fluids. Approval from competent regulatory agencies, such as the U.S. FDA or the EMA, is required before such devices can be marketed or used in clinical settings.

In the United States, the FDA classifies most FET biosensors used for medical diagnostics as Class II medical devices, which carry a moderate risk and require special regulatory controls. Devices intended for home-based or point-of-care use generally follow the 510(k) premarket notification pathway, in which manufacturers must demonstrate that their new product is substantially equivalent to an existing approved device [85]. For higher-risk or novel biosensors, the Premarket Approval (PMA) process may be required, which may involve more comprehensive clinical evidence.

In the European Union, FET biosensors fall under either the Medical Device Regulation (MDR 2017/745) or the In Vitro Diagnostic Regulation (IVDR 2017/746), depending on their intended use. To obtain a CE mark, manufacturers must prove that the device meets essential safety and performance standards, which are verified by a notified body. Devices are classified into risk categories (A–D), and FET biosensors are generally categorized as Class B or C, requiring analytical validation and clinical performance studies before approval. Compliance also includes adherence to ISO 13485, the international standard for quality management systems in medical device manufacturing.

Even after approval, post-market surveillance (PMS) remains mandatory under regulatory oversight. PMS involves systematic collection and analysis of data on device performance, safety incidents, and user feedback once the biosensor is commercially available. Reports of device malfunction, inaccurate readings, or adverse events are analyzed to identify and correct potential problems. In the European Union, manufacturers must maintain a Post-Market Surveillance Plan (PMSP) and submit regular Periodic Safety Update Reports (PSUR) to regulatory authorities. For high-risk biosensors, additional Post-Market Clinical Follow-Up (PMCF) studies are often required to confirm ongoing clinical safety and effectiveness. Similarly, the FDA mandates Medical Device Reporting (MDR) to track adverse events and recalls in the United States. Post-market monitoring also encompasses data from clinicians, patients, and digital sources. Modern FET biosensors often include wireless connectivity and software components that transmit performance logs to secure databases. This enables real-time oversight of device behavior and facilitates continuous quality improvement.

2.5.6   *Future Perspectives*

The future of FET-based biosensors in medicine and biotechnology is exceptionally promising. Their unique combination of high sensitivity, fast response time, and potential for miniaturization positions them as key technologies for next-generation diagnostics and monitoring systems. Continuous advances in materials science, nanotechnology, and electronic engineering are expanding their capabilities, enabling more sophisticated and versatile biosensing applications.

In clinical practice, FET biosensors are expected to become central to continuous health monitoring through wearable and implantable devices. These systems can measure physiological parameters in real time, allowing early detection of abnormalities and continuous disease management. For patients with chronic conditions such as diabetes, cardiovascular disorders, or neurodegenerative diseases, such devices offer the possibility of round-the-clock monitoring without invasive procedures [86]. The integration of FET biosensors into medical implants and portable diagnostic tools will help bridge the gap between clinical laboratories and personalized healthcare.

A significant future direction lies in the development of **multiplexed biosensors,** capable of detecting several biomarkers simultaneously. By analyzing complex biological samples for multiple indicators of disease, these systems will provide more accurate diagnostic information and reduce the time required for clinical decision-making. Lab-on-a-chip platforms, which integrate FET biosensors with microfluidic systems, are already paving the way for compact, automated diagnostic devices that require only microliters of biological fluid to deliver rapid and precise results. Another major trend is the use of advanced nanomaterials, such as graphene, molybdenum disulfide (MoS_2), and carbon nanotubes. These materials possess remarkable electrical and chemical properties that enhance the sensitivity, selectivity, and stability of FET sensors. For instance, graphene's large surface area and high conductivity make it an ideal channel material for detecting even trace amounts of biomolecules. Similarly, integrating hybrid nanomaterial composites can improve device durability and extend operational life under physiological conditions.

The concept of personalized medicine is also closely tied to the evolution of FET biosensors. Because these devices can measure specific biochemical changes in individual patients, they enable clinicians to tailor treatment strategies based on real-time physiological feedback. Such personalization helps optimize therapy effectiveness, minimize side effects, and support proactive healthcare rather than reactive intervention [87]. Beyond medical diagnostics, FET biosensors are expected to play transformative roles in other fields such as environmental monitoring, food safety, and biotechnology. They can detect contaminants, toxins, or pathogens in air, water, and food with exceptional accuracy, supporting public health and industrial safety. Moreover, their integration into industrial bioprocesses can enable precise control of fermentation, enzymatic reactions, and other biochemical operations (Fig. 2.28).

Ongoing advances in sensor miniaturization and data connectivity will further promote the widespread use of FET biosensors. Their compatibility with wireless systems, smartphones, and Internet of Things (IoT) platforms enables seamless data transfer, remote monitoring, and integration with digital health infrastructures. This

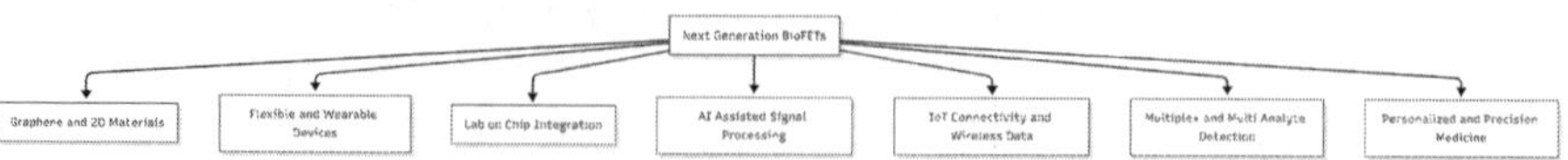

Fig. 2.28 Emerging directions in FET biosensing

shift toward connected biosensing networks marks a new era of proactive, continuous, and data-driven healthcare.

2.6 Immunosensors

Immunosensors are advanced analytical devices that merge the selectivity of immunological reactions with the precision of modern transduction technologies to detect and measure specific biomolecules. They rely on the highly specific interaction between antibodies and antigens, enabling the accurate identification of a wide range of biological targets, including proteins, pathogens, and disease-related biomarkers [88]. By combining biological recognition with sensitive signal detection, immunosensors have transformed diagnostic science, offering fast, accurate, and reliable detection methods that are essential for early disease diagnosis, patient monitoring, and therapeutic management (Fig. 2.29).

The working principle of an immunosensor is based on the formation of an **immunocomplex,** in which an antibody binds specifically to its corresponding antigen. This antigen–antibody interaction produces a measurable change that can be captured and quantified by a transducer. Depending on the design, the transducer may operate through electrochemical, optical, or piezoelectric mechanisms, each influencing the sensor's performance characteristics, including sensitivity, selectivity, and response time. Among these options, electrochemical immunosensors have become particularly prominent due to their exceptional sensitivity, ease of miniaturization, and compatibility with portable platforms—qualities that make them well-suited for point-of-care testing.

The origin of immunosensor technology dates back to the 1970s, when researchers began adapting principles from **enzyme-linked immunosorbent assays (ELISA)** to develop devices capable of real-time detection. Over subsequent decades, advances in materials science and nanotechnology revolutionized the field. The integration of nanomaterials, such as gold nanoparticles, carbon nanotubes, and graphene, greatly enhanced surface conductivity and increased the active surface area, thereby improving signal amplification and lowering detection limits. As a result, immunosensors now extend beyond traditional clinical diagnostics into environmental monitoring, food safety, and biodefense.

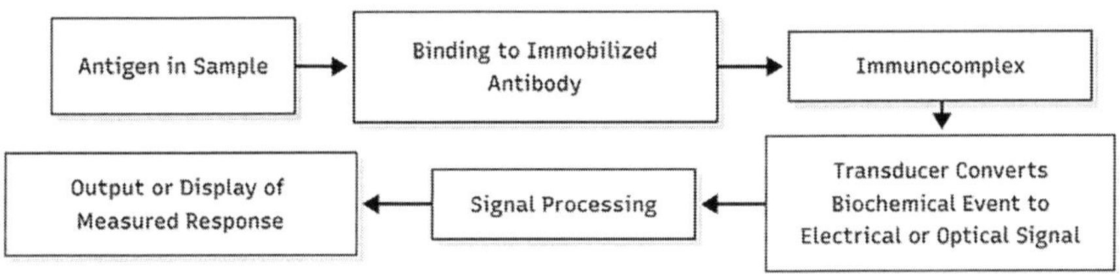

Fig. 2.29 Basic principle of an immunosensor

130
2 Types of Biosensors

In medicine, immunosensors are increasingly important for detecting cancer biomarkers, infectious agents, and therapeutic drug levels. Their ability to measure analytes at trace concentrations enables early-stage diagnosis, which is critical for successful treatment and disease management [89]. Rapid immunosensor-based detection of viral antigens or antibodies has also proven invaluable for managing infectious disease outbreaks, providing fast, on-site diagnostic results. Moreover, the portability and ease of use of modern immunosensors make them accessible tools for point-of-care and field testing, improving healthcare availability in remote or resource-limited regions.

Despite remarkable progress, several challenges persist. Issues such as non-specific binding, signal interference, and the need for rigorous validation continue to shape ongoing research and development. Additionally, adherence to strict regulatory and safety standards remains a prerequisite for clinical implementation. Nevertheless, the continuous refinement of immunosensor technology, through innovations in nanomaterials, signal processing, and biointerface engineering, promises even greater diagnostic capability and broader applicability in the years ahead.

2.6.1 History

The development of immunosensors is closely linked to the broader evolution of biosensing technologies and advances in immunology with Clark's pioneering work laid the foundation for modern biosensors, including immunosensors (Fig. 2.30).

The concept of immunosensors began to take shape during the 1970s as researchers recognized the potential of combining immunological specificity with real-time signal transduction. A major milestone during this era was the introduction of **ELISA** which utilized antibodies immobilized on solid supports to selectively bind target antigens. The ensuing enzymatic reactions produced measurable signals that reflected the analyte's presence and concentration. ELISA highlighted the precision and sensitivity of antibody–antigen interactions and inspired scientists to develop sensor systems that translate these interactions into continuous electrical or optical outputs.

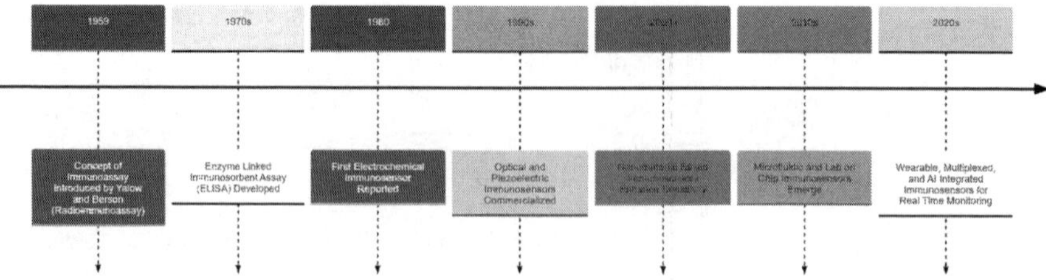

Fig. 2.30 Timeline of immunosensor evolution

During the 1980s and 1990s, rapid progress in miniaturization and microelectronics enabled the development of integrated immunosensing systems. Electrochemical immunosensors became especially prominent, converting antigen–antibody binding events into electrical signals that could be measured directly. Researchers such as Wang and colleagues demonstrated that electrochemical detection methods, including amperometry, potentiometry, and impedance spectroscopy, offered remarkable speed and sensitivity, making them ideal for clinical and point-of-care applications [90]. These developments not only advanced the performance of immunosensors but also set the stage for portable diagnostic platforms that could deliver results outside of conventional laboratories.

The early 2000s marked a transformative period marked by the integration of nanotechnology. Nanomaterials such as gold nanoparticles, carbon nanotubes, and graphene were incorporated into immunosensor designs, dramatically increasing surface area and enhancing electron transfer processes. This innovation enabled the detection of biomolecules at previously unattainable concentrations, expanding the use of immunosensors beyond clinical diagnostics into environmental monitoring, food safety, and security applications. Nanostructured materials also improved sensor stability and biocompatibility, further enhancing their performance and reliability.

In recent years, the field has continued to evolve through the convergence of biosensing, materials science, and data analytics. The integration of AI and ML has opened new possibilities for advanced data interpretation, improving both diagnostic precision and predictive capability. Portable and user-friendly immunosensor systems are now being developed for use in hospitals, clinics, and even remote or field settings. These modern devices enable fast, accurate measurements while minimizing the need for specialized equipment or trained personnel.

Despite these significant advancements, several challenges remain central to the ongoing development of immunosensors. Ensuring consistent analytical performance, maintaining stability in complex biological matrices, and addressing issues such as non-specific adsorption are active areas of research. Furthermore, regulatory validation and compliance remain essential steps in transitioning new immunosensor technologies into clinical practice.

The history of immunosensors thus reflects a continual evolution, from early enzyme-based electrodes to highly sophisticated nanomaterial-enhanced systems capable of real-time, high-precision detection [91]. This progression underscores the interdisciplinary nature of the field, merging chemistry, biology, physics, and engineering to create technologies that are now indispensable in modern diagnostics and public health.

2.6.2 Technical Characteristics

Immunosensors are sophisticated analytical systems that integrate biological recognition mechanisms with physicochemical signal transduction to detect and quantify specific analytes. Their technical characteristics determine how effectively they

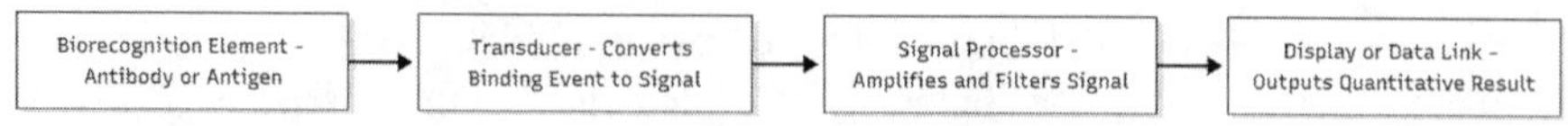

Fig. 2.31 Functional block diagram of an immunosensor

perform, influencing reliability, accuracy, and suitability for clinical or environmental use. These characteristics encompass both the hardware and software components, as well as key performance indicators that define the sensor's analytical behavior (Fig. 2.31).

Hardware

The hardware of an immunosensor typically includes three primary elements: a biorecognition component, a transducer, and a signal-processing unit. The biorecognition component, usually composed of antibodies or antigens, is responsible for ensuring specificity by binding selectively to the target analyte. This molecular recognition event underlies the sensor's operation, translating a biological interaction into a physical or chemical change. The transducer converts this binding event into a measurable signal. Depending on the detection method, the signal can be electrochemical, optical, or piezoelectric [91]. Electrochemical transducers are among the most commonly used because of their high sensitivity, short response time, and compatibility with miniaturized devices. Optical transducers detect changes in fluorescence, absorbance, or refractive index, while piezoelectric transducers measure shifts in mass or resonance frequency resulting from antigen–antibody binding (Table 2.19).

The signal-processing unit amplifies, filters, and digitizes the raw signal generated by the transducer. This stage often includes analog-to-digital converters and microprocessors that apply algorithms to reduce background noise and enhance measurement precision. Through this process, weak electrical or optical signals are transformed into stable, interpretable outputs that can be displayed numerically or graphically. The hardware of an immunosensor serves as the foundation of its analytical performance, integrating biological recognition elements with physical components that generate, process, and transmit measurable signals. Each component must function harmoniously to ensure precision, stability, and responsiveness in detecting target analytes.

At the heart of every immunosensor is the **biorecognition element**, which provides the device's essential selectivity. This element, most often an antibody or antigen, is responsible for binding specifically to the analyte of interest. The choice of biorecognition molecule is a critical design consideration, as it directly affects the sensor's specificity, sensitivity, and detection limits. Antibodies with high binding affinity are typically selected to ensure the reliable detection of low-abundance targets.

Various types of recognition elements can be employed depending on the intended application [92]:

- **Antibodies** are the most common and well-established recognition molecules, known for their exceptional specificity toward antigens. Both monoclonal and polyclonal antibodies are used, chosen based on desired selectivity and binding kinetics.

Table 2.19 Common transducer types

Type	Detected property	Output signal	Typical use
Electrochemical	Redox/charge	Current/potential	Blood analytes
Optical	Fluorescence/RI	Intensity/angle	Kinetic binding
Piezoelectric	Mass/elasticity	Frequency	Food/environment
Thermometric	Heat change	Temperature	Low-resource assays

- **Antigens** are utilized in reverse immunoassays when antibodies serve as the target analytes.
- **Aptamers**, synthetic single-stranded DNA or RNA sequences, can bind a wide variety of targets with high affinity. They offer greater stability, cost-effectiveness, and reusability than antibodies.
- **Peptides** are short amino acid chains that mimic antibody-binding sites, providing selectivity while allowing easier synthesis and modification.
- **Receptors**, whether natural or engineered, can recognize specific ligands and be immobilized on sensor surfaces to enable selective detection.
- **Molecularly imprinted polymers (MIPs)** are synthetic recognition materials designed to replicate natural binding sites of biomolecules, combining robustness, reusability, and high stability.

Following the biorecognition event, the transducer converts the biochemical interaction into a measurable signal. Several types of transducers are employed in immunosensors [93]:

- **Electrochemical transducers** detect changes in current, potential, or impedance resulting from antigen–antibody binding. They are highly sensitive, rapid, and easily miniaturized, making them ideal for point-of-care diagnostics.
- **Optical transducers** rely on variations in optical properties, such as fluorescence, absorbance, or refractive index, that occur when immunocomplexes form. They are valued for their high sensitivity and real-time monitoring capabilities.
- **Piezoelectric transducers** exploit the piezoelectric effect to measure changes in mass or mechanical properties on the sensor surface. These label-free systems are particularly effective for detecting small molecules and dynamic binding events.

Once a signal is generated, it is processed through a signal-processing unit, which amplifies, filters, and digitizes the output. This unit typically consists of electronic circuits, analog-to-digital converters (ADCs), and microprocessors that apply mathematical algorithms to enhance signal clarity. Amplification ensures weak electrical or optical signals are measurable, while digital conversion allows the data to be further analyzed, displayed, or transmitted.

Software

The software integrated within immunosensors plays a pivotal role in managing data acquisition, calibration, analysis, and interpretation. Advanced algorithms enable real time monitoring and correction for environmental fluctuations, temperature variations, or sensor drift. Modern immunosensor platforms often incorporate digital signal-processing techniques that filter out unwanted interference and improve the signal-to-noise ratio, enabling accurate detection of even low-concentration analytes. In more recent designs, ML and statistical modeling tools have been introduced to analyze complex, multidimensional datasets generated during immunoassays. These computational approaches enhance detection accuracy by identifying patterns, nonlinear relationships, and subtle fluctuations that traditional methods may overlook. As a result, immunosensors have evolved from simple detection devices into intelligent analytical systems capable of performing predictive diagnostics and trend analysis.

Several key parameters define an immunosensor's performance and determine its effectiveness in real-world applications. Sensitivity measures the device's ability to detect very low concentrations of an analyte, a crucial factor for early disease diagnosis and environmental monitoring [94]. Specificity reflects the sensor's capacity to recognize the target analyte exclusively, minimizing interference from structurally similar compounds. Response time is the time it takes for the sensor to generate a measurable signal after sample introduction, which is especially critical in time-sensitive clinical situations. Other important metrics include dynamic range, representing the span of analyte concentrations that can be accurately measured, and stability, which indicates the sensor's ability to maintain consistent performance over repeated uses or extended operation. Long-term reproducibility is also essential for ensuring that identical samples yield consistent results under similar conditions.

The software components of immunosensors are central to their analytical capability, transforming raw signals into meaningful diagnostic information. As immunosensors become increasingly complex, incorporating multiple transducers and generating vast quantities of data, sophisticated software systems are essential for managing calibration, data acquisition, processing, and interpretation.

Modern immunosensor software performs several critical functions that directly influence the precision and reliability of measurements:

- Calibration ensures accuracy by compensating for signal fluctuations caused by environmental conditions, sensor aging, or drift. Dynamic calibration routines automatically adjust response parameters, ensuring consistent performance even under variable conditions.
- Data acquisition and preprocessing involve collecting raw signals from the transducer and refining them to remove noise or irrelevant background information. Advanced filtering methods, such as wavelet transforms, moving average filters, and baseline correction, enhance the clarity of the recorded signal, making it suitable for further quantitative analysis.
- Normalization and scaling standardize data across multiple measurements or sensor batches, ensuring that results remain comparable and reproducible.

Once preprocessing is complete, the data are subjected to feature extraction, during which key parameters, such as peak amplitude, signal decay rate, and frequency components, are identified and analyzed. These features serve as input to computational algorithms that determine analyte concentration or classify a sample's biological state.

Recent developments have introduced ML and AI into immunosensor software frameworks [95]. These tools provide advanced analytical power beyond traditional calibration curves or threshold-based detection. ML models can recognize subtle signal variations, nonlinear correlations, and complex relationships within biosensor data, leading to more accurate and robust detection outcomes (Table 2.20).

Depending on the application, different ML approaches may be employed [96]:

- **Supervised learning models**—such as Random Forests, Support Vector Regression (SVR), and Neural Networks—are trained using labeled datasets to predict analyte concentrations or classify disease states.
- **Unsupervised learning algorithms**, including k-means and hierarchical clustering, automatically group similar signal patterns, aiding biomarker discovery and patient stratification.
- **Dimensionality reduction techniques**, such as Principal Component Analysis (PCA) or t-distributed Stochastic Neighbor Embedding (t-SNE), allow visualization of complex, high-dimensional datasets to identify trends and hidden structures.
- **Deep learning architectures**, including Convolutional Neural Networks (CNNs) and Recurrent Neural Networks (RNNs), are particularly effective for interpreting time-series or spectral data and are increasingly applied in wearable or continuous monitoring systems.

These computational techniques have expanded the diagnostic potential of immunosensors far beyond simple detection. For example, in early disease diagnostics, ML enhances the identification of low-abundance biomarkers that traditional methods might overlook. In multiplexed immunosensing, where several biomarkers are measured simultaneously, AI-based analysis can decode overlapping signals, ensuring precise quantification of each analyte [97]. Real-time systems benefit from adaptive algorithms that continuously process streaming data and dynamically adjust responses, enabling their use in intensive care monitoring and personalized healthcare.

Key analytical parameters, such as sensitivity, specificity, response time, dynamic range, stability, and reproducibility, are also managed and optimized using software algorithms. Sensitivity determines the lowest detectable analyte concentration, while specificity ensures that only the intended target is measured without

Table 2.20 Software functions and algorithms

Function	Technique	Purpose
Baseline correction	Moving average/wavelet	Remove drift
Feature extraction	Peak detection/FFT	Quantify signal
Classification	SVM/Random Forest	Identify analyte
Regression	Neural network	Estimate concentration
Visualization	PCA/Dashboard	Interpret trends

cross-reactivity. Response time quantifies how quickly the system delivers results, and stability indicates its consistency over repeated cycles. Together, these parameters define the overall analytical robustness of the immunosensor.

The integration of advanced data analytics and ML has transformed immunosensors into intelligent diagnostic systems. Rather than serving solely as detection tools, they now act as digital analytical platforms capable of recognizing patterns, predicting outcomes, and guiding medical decisions. As computational capabilities continue to evolve, software will remain the defining component that bridges biological recognition with actionable insight in next-generation biosensing technologies.

2.6.3 Types of Devices

Immunosensors can be categorized based on their transduction mechanisms and detection formats. Each device type offers unique advantages depending on the required sensitivity, specificity, portability, and intended application. The four primary categories include electrochemical, optical, piezoelectric, and thermometric immunosensors [98]. These systems differ in how they convert biological recognition events into measurable signals but share the same fundamental principle of antibody–antigen interaction (Fig. 2.32).

Electrochemical immunosensors are among the most widely adopted due to their exceptional sensitivity, compact design, and compatibility with low-cost, miniaturized platforms. These sensors measure electrical signals generated during immunochemical reactions and are particularly suitable for point-of-care diagnostics [99]. They can be subdivided into several categories according to the specific electrochemical technique employed:

- **Amperometric immunosensors** measure the current generated by the oxidation or reduction of electroactive species involved in the immunoreaction. The generated current is proportional to the concentration of the target analyte. These sensors are commonly used for detecting biomarkers such as carcinoembryonic antigen (CEA) and prostate-specific antigen (PSA) in cancer diagnostics.
- **Potentiometric immunosensors** detect changes in electrode potential (voltage) at the electrode surface as antigen–antibody binding occurs. The resulting potential shift correlates with analyte concentration. Their simplicity, low cost, and

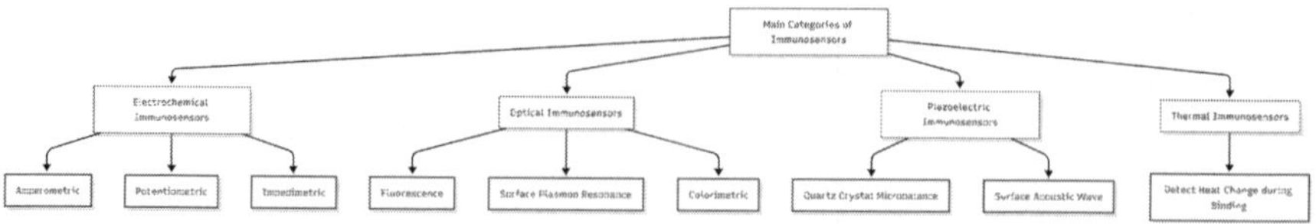

Fig. 2.32 Main categories of immunosensors

energy efficiency make them highly suitable for portable and disposable testing devices, including hormone and therapeutic drug detection.

- **Impedimetric immunosensors** measure variations in impedance at the electrode interface due to biomolecular binding. Because they do not require labeling agents, these sensors provide label-free detection and are highly sensitive to small changes in the interfacial environment. They are frequently used for detecting infectious agents and toxins.
- **Voltammetric immunosensors** apply controlled voltage sweeps, such as cyclic voltammetry (CV) or differential pulse voltammetry (DPV), to record current responses that reveal the redox properties of target molecules. They are advantageous for multiplexed detection, enabling simultaneous monitoring of multiple analytes in clinical and food-safety applications (Table 2.21).
- **Optical immunosensors** detect antigen–antibody interactions by monitoring changes in optical signals, including fluorescence, absorbance, and refractive index. Their capacity for real-time, label-free monitoring and high sensitivity makes them valuable tools in medical diagnostics, environmental analysis, and pharmaceutical research [100].

The main subtypes include:

- **Fluorescent immunosensors**, which employ fluorescent tags attached to antibodies or antigens. The binding of the analyte triggers the emission of light at a specific wavelength, which can be quantified to determine the analyte concentration. These sensors are widely used for early detection of cancer biomarkers and infectious agents.
- **SPR immunosensors**, which measure refractive index changes at a metal surface (typically gold) as biomolecules bind. SPR enables real-time observation of binding kinetics without labeling, providing valuable insights into drug discovery and biomolecular interactions.
- **Colorimetric immunosensors**, which produce visible color changes upon target binding. These systems can be analyzed by eye or with a spectrophotometer and are ideal for rapid point-of-care or field testing, such as detecting foodborne pathogens and environmental toxins (Table 2.22).

Optical immunosensors are valued for their non-destructive nature, enabling repeatable and continuous measurements with minimal sample preparation. **Piezoelectric and thermometric immunosensors** operate based on physical property changes, mass, mechanical resonance, or heat, arising from antigen–antibody binding. These devices are especially suited for label-free and quantitative analysis of molecular

Table 2.21 Electrochemical immunosensor subtypes

Subtype	Measured parameter	Label	Example biomarker
Amperometric	Current	Enzyme-labeled	PSA, CEA
Potentiometric	Voltage	Label-free	Hormones
Impedimetric	Impedance	Label-free	Bacterial antigens
Voltammetric	Current vs voltage	Label-based/free	Multi-analyte panels

Table 2.22 Optical immunosensor methods

Type	Signal	Label requirement	Sensitivity	Typical field
Fluorescent	Light emission	Yes	10^{-12} M	Cancer diagnostics
SPR	Refractive index	No	10^{-9} M	Drug discovery
Colorimetric	Visible color	Optional	10^{-6} M	Food safety

interactions [101]. **QCM immunosensors** measure frequency shifts in a vibrating quartz crystal as analyte molecules bind to its surface. The magnitude of the frequency change directly corresponds to the mass of the bound analyte, providing quantitative information. QCM sensors are extensively used for environmental monitoring and food safety testing. **SAW immunosensors** employ acoustic waves that travel across a piezoelectric substrate. The propagation characteristics of these waves change upon biomolecular binding, allowing highly sensitive detection of small analytes in clinical or environmental samples. **Thermometric (calorimetric) immunosensors** detect temperature changes resulting from exothermic or endothermic reactions during antigen–antibody interactions. These systems are cost-effective, easy to operate, and suitable for detecting a broad range of biomolecules in resource-limited settings. Although less common than electrochemical and optical variants, these sensors offer distinct advantages, including label-free operation, direct mass measurement, and the ability to function in complex sample matrices.

2.6.4   Clinical Applications

Immunosensors have become indispensable tools in modern clinical diagnostics, offering rapid, sensitive, and highly specific detection of disease biomarkers. Their ability to deliver real-time or near-real-time results makes them essential in hospital laboratories, emergency settings, and point-of-care applications where timely clinical decisions are crucial. These devices enable early diagnosis, continuous disease monitoring, and personalized therapeutic management, significantly improving the quality and efficiency of patient care.

The primary use of immunosensors in clinical medicine is the detection of biomarkers associated with diseases such as cancer, infectious disorders, and autoimmune conditions. By combining the selectivity of antibody–antigen interactions with advanced signal transduction methods, immunosensors can identify extremely low concentrations of target molecules in biological samples, providing valuable diagnostic information [102].

Cancer biomarkers are among the most studied targets for immunosensor-based assays. Tumor markers such as carcinoembryonic antigen (CEA), prostate-specific antigen (PSA), and alpha-fetoprotein (AFP) are routinely analyzed in oncology. Electrochemical immunosensors capable of detecting trace levels of these proteins in serum samples allow early diagnosis, monitoring of treatment response, and assessment of disease recurrence. Because early detection often determines patient survival, these devices play a critical role in preventive oncology and therapy management.

In **infectious disease diagnostics**, immunosensors provide rapid and accurate detection of pathogens or host antibodies. During the COVID-19 pandemic, for example, electrochemical and optical immunosensors were used to identify viral antigens or antibodies within minutes—far faster than conventional laboratory-based methods. Such technologies are invaluable in outbreak control, where immediate diagnosis can help isolate cases, initiate treatment, and prevent disease spread.

Autoimmune disorders represent another major area where immunosensors have proven useful. These conditions arise when the immune system mistakenly targets the body's own tissues. Biomarkers such as anti-nuclear antibodies (ANA) and rheumatoid factor (RF) can be efficiently measured using immunosensors, enabling clinicians to diagnose and monitor diseases such as systemic lupus erythematosus and rheumatoid arthritis [103]. The speed and accuracy of these measurements enable more precise therapy adjustments and improved long-term management.

Beyond diagnosis, immunosensors are valuable tools for tracking disease progression and assessing treatment efficacy. Their high sensitivity allows for longitudinal monitoring of biomarker levels, providing clinicians with real-time insight into therapeutic outcomes and patient status.

Therapeutic drug monitoring (TDM) is one important application. Maintaining optimal drug concentrations is essential for efficacy and safety, particularly for medications with narrow therapeutic windows. Immunosensors can measure drug levels directly in patient samples, helping ensure appropriate dosing. For instance, they are commonly used to monitor immunosuppressant levels in organ transplant recipients, minimizing the risk of rejection or toxicity.

Immunosensors are also used for **tracking disease progression**, where continuous or periodic biomarker measurements provide early indications of relapse or complications. In oncology, monitoring tumor marker concentrations helps evaluate treatment effectiveness and detect recurrence. Similarly, in chronic viral infections such as HIV, immunosensors can track viral load and immune response, guiding therapy adjustments and improving patient prognosis. The integration of immunosensors into point-of-care (POC) devices has revolutionized clinical testing by enabling diagnostics outside of centralized laboratories. POC immunosensors are compact, portable, and user-friendly, enabling rapid diagnosis at the bedside, in outpatient clinics, and even in remote, resource-limited settings [104].

Bedside testing using immunosensors allows clinicians to obtain immediate diagnostic information without waiting for laboratory confirmation. For example, cardiac biomarker sensors can identify troponin or creatine kinase levels in patients presenting with chest pain, facilitating prompt diagnosis of myocardial infarction and early intervention. Remote monitoring is another emerging application enabled by wearable or portable immunosensors. These devices can continuously track biomarkers for diabetes, cardiovascular disease, or inflammation, and transmit data wirelessly to healthcare providers. Such systems support personalized medicine by enabling real-time feedback, early detection of complications, and timely adjustments to treatment. Remote immunosensor monitoring also empowers patients to take an active role in managing chronic illnesses, improving adherence, and long-term outcomes.

2.6.5   Regulatory Considerations

The integration of immunosensors into clinical practice requires strict adherence to regulatory and quality standards that ensure their safety, efficacy, and reliability. Because these devices directly influence diagnostic and therapeutic decisions, regulatory oversight is essential at every stage, from design and preclinical testing to post-market surveillance. Agencies such as the U.S. FDA and the EMA define comprehensive frameworks governing the development, evaluation, and approval of medical devices.

Immunosensors are classified as medical devices, and their regulatory pathway depends on their intended use and the risk to patients. In the United States, the FDA categorizes devices into three classes [105]:

- Class I (low-risk): Subject to general controls with minimal regulatory requirements. Most Class I devices are exempt from premarket notification.
- Class II (moderate-risk): Requires premarket notification through the 510(k) process, which demonstrates that the new device is substantially equivalent to an already approved (predicate) device.
- Class III (high-risk): Requires premarket approval (PMA), the most rigorous pathway, including extensive safety and performance data, often from clinical trials.

In the European Union, immunosensors fall under the Medical Device Regulation (MDR 2017/745) or the In Vitro Diagnostic Regulation (IVDR 2017/746). Devices are classified by risk level from Class A (lowest risk) to Class D (highest risk). Most diagnostic immunosensors fall within Class B or C, requiring conformity assessments, clinical validation, and the CE marking, which certifies compliance with essential safety and performance standards.

Before any immunosensor reaches the market, it must undergo a series of preclinical and clinical evaluations to establish its analytical validity, clinical utility, and safety.

Preclinical studies involve laboratory-based evaluations of analytical performance, including sensitivity, specificity, accuracy, and precision. These studies assess the sensor's ability to reliably detect the target analyte. Clinical trials are required for higher-risk devices (typically Class II and III). Conducted in accordance with Good Clinical Practice (GCP) guidelines, they assess the immunosensor's diagnostic accuracy and usability in real-world patient populations, ensuring consistent performance under clinical conditions.

As the field advances, harmonization of global regulatory standards has become increasingly important. Collaborative efforts between international regulatory bodies, manufacturers, and researchers are essential to streamline approval processes while maintaining patient safety and promoting innovation.

After regulatory approval, ongoing post-market surveillance (PMS) is required to monitor device performance and detect potential safety issues under real-world conditions.

Manufacturers must establish PMS systems that [106]:

- Collect data on device malfunctions, false readings, and adverse events.
- Record feedback from clinicians and patients regarding usability and performance.
- Track software updates and hardware modifications that may affect analytical accuracy.
- Submit Periodic Safety Update Reports (PSURs) summarizing safety findings to regulatory authorities.

For higher-risk immunosensors, Post-Market Clinical Follow-Up (PMCF) studies may be required to validate continued clinical performance over time. These measures ensure that devices remain safe, effective, and aligned with evolving clinical standards.

2.6.6 Future Perspectives

The field of immunosensors is rapidly progressing, driven by continual advances in materials science, nanotechnology, data analytics, and biomedical engineering. These developments are redefining how diseases are detected, monitored, and managed, bringing diagnostics closer to patients and enabling personalized, predictive healthcare. As the demand for faster, more reliable, and decentralized testing grows, immunosensors are positioned to play an increasingly prominent role across clinical, environmental, and industrial domains (Fig. 2.33).

A primary goal in the next generation of immunosensor development is to enhance both sensitivity and specificity, enabling the detection of ultralow analyte concentrations and improved discrimination between closely related biomolecules. Emerging research focuses on integrating nanomaterials, such as gold nanoparticles, carbon nanotubes, graphene, and metal–organic frameworks (MOFs). These materials provide larger active surface areas, superior electrical conductivity, and unique optical properties that amplify signal responses from antigen–antibody interactions.

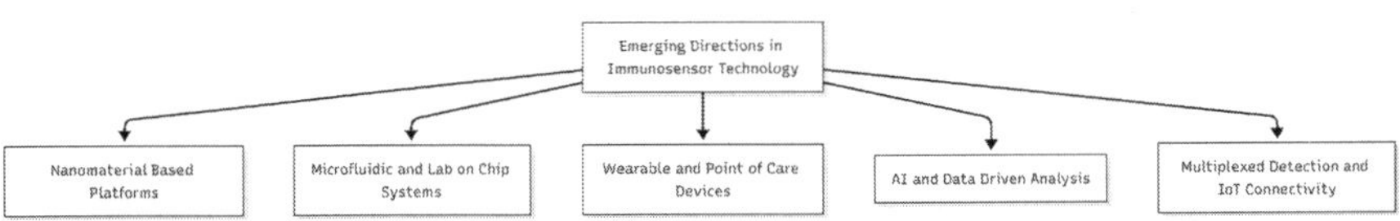

Fig. 2.33 Emerging directions in immunosensor technology

The use of **hybrid nanostructures** and **functionalized composite materials** is expected to further improve signal transduction and minimize background noise. Additionally, signal amplification strategies, including enzymatic catalysis, redox cycling, and molecular beacon systems, are being optimized to detect trace levels of biomarkers [107]. Such advancements are essential for early disease diagnosis, where biomarker concentrations are often exceedingly low.

Multiplexing technologies represent another promising direction, enabling simultaneous detection of multiple biomarkers within a single assay. This approach allows clinicians to construct comprehensive biochemical profiles, offering a more holistic understanding of disease states and therapeutic responses.

The future of immunosensors is closely tied to their **integration with digital health platforms**, wearable technologies, and POC devices. The ongoing miniaturization of sensor systems and the expansion of wireless communication capabilities have enabled the development of portable, user-friendly diagnostic devices that deliver laboratory-quality results beyond traditional healthcare facilities. Upcoming generations of immunosensors are expected to feature real-time connectivity through Bluetooth, Wi-Fi, or cellular networks, enabling seamless transmission of results to electronic health records (EHRs) or mobile health applications [108]. This interconnectivity will enhance telemedicine services by allowing physicians to monitor patients remotely and respond promptly to physiological changes. ML and AI will play an increasingly important role in data interpretation, enabling automatic pattern recognition, trend analysis, and anomaly detection from complex biosensor datasets. By linking biosensor readings to predictive models, AI-driven analysis can forecast disease progression or therapeutic response before clinical symptoms manifest.

The movement toward personalized medicine is one of the most transformative trends shaping the future of immunosensors. As individual genetic and metabolic variability becomes better understood, diagnostic technologies are being adapted to tailor treatment strategies based on patient-specific biomarker profiles. Immunosensors will play a pivotal role in both biomarker discovery and individualized monitoring. By detecting specific proteins, metabolites, or antibodies that vary between patients, these devices can support customized therapy plans, optimize drug dosing, and minimize adverse effects [109]. Real-time immunosensor data can provide clinicians with immediate feedback on therapeutic efficacy, enabling dynamic adjustment of medication regimens. For instance, tracking inflammatory cytokines or drug metabolites using wearable immunosensors could enable clinicians to modify treatment before complications arise.

The potential applications of immunosensors extend well beyond clinical diagnostics. Their high sensitivity and selectivity make them valuable tools for environmental monitoring, food safety, and biodefense. In environmental science, immunosensors can rapidly detect pollutants, toxins, and pathogens in water, soil, and air. The ability to conduct on-site testing without extensive sample preparation is particularly useful for environmental protection agencies and industries responsible for waste management and contamination control. In the food industry, immunosensors can accurately detect allergens, pathogens, and spoilage indicators, thereby improving food safety and quality control. Additionally, their portability allows for real-time analysis during food production and distribution. In biodefense and public safety, immunosensors are being developed to detect biological warfare agents and emerging infectious pathogens [110]. The integration of these devices into automated surveillance systems could provide early warning of biological threats, strengthening public health preparedness. As sustainability and environmental accountability become global priorities, immunosensors will play an increasingly important role in ensuring ecological integrity and consumer safety through rapid, accurate detection technologies.

With the worldwide commercialization of immunosensors, post-market monitoring has become a key component of regulatory and industrial strategy. Regulatory agencies across major markets have implemented systems to track device safety and performance following approval. In the United States, the FDA utilizes the Manufacturer and User Facility Device Experience (MAUDE) database and the MedSun network to collect post-market data on device performance and adverse events. In the European Union, the EudraVigilance system and mandatory Post-Market Clinical Follow-Up (PMCF) studies ensure continuous monitoring of safety and effectiveness. Many countries are adopting Unique Device Identification (UDI) systems to improve traceability by linking manufacturing data to clinical outcomes. Additionally, real-world evidence derived from electronic health records and insurance databases is increasingly used to assess device reliability in diverse populations. Manufacturers are now required to submit Periodic Safety Update Reports (PSURs) and, for high-risk devices, conduct targeted post-approval studies. These surveillance strategies strengthen regulatory confidence and ensure long-term clinical reliability, especially as immunosensors become more complex and interconnected.

References

1. Kim J, Jeong J, Ko SH. Electrochemical biosensors for point-of-care testing. Bio-Des Manuf. 2024;7(4):548–65.
2. Sumitha MS, Xavier TS. Recent advances in electrochemical biosensors—a brief review. Hybrid Adv. 2023;2:100023.
3. Cui H, Xin X, Su J, Song S. Research progress of electrochemical biosensors for disease detection in China: a review. Biosensors. 2025;15(4):231.
4. Wachholz D Jr, Deroco PB, Hryniewicz BM, Kubota LT. Strategies for electrochemical point-of-care biosensors. Annu Rev Anal Chem. 2025;18
5. Wang K, Lin X, Zhang M, Li Y, Luo C, Wu J. Review of electrochemical biosensors for food-safety detection. Biosensors. 2022;12(11):959.
6. Zhao Z, Cao J, Zhu B, Li X, Zhou L, Su B. Recent advances in MXene-based electrochemical sensors. Biosensors. 2025;15(2):107.
7. DeVoe E, Andreescu S. Catalytic electrochemical biosensors for dopamine: design, performance, and healthcare applications. ECS Sens Plus. 2024;3(2):020601.
8. Sardini E, Serpelloni M, Tonello S. Printed electrochemical biosensors: opportunities and metrological challenges. Biosensors. 2020;10(11):166.

9. Guo L, Zhao Y, Huang Q, Huang J, Tao Y, Chen J, et al. Electrochemical protein biosensors for disease-marker detection: progress and opportunities. Microsyst Nanoeng. 2024;10(1):65.

10. Manoharan Nair Sudha Kumari S, Thankappan Suryabai X. Sensing the future—frontiers in biosensors: classifications, principles, and recent advances. ACS Omega. 2024;9(50):48918–87.

11. Jung HH, Lee H, Yea J, Jang KI. Wearable electrochemical sensors for real-time monitoring in diabetes mellitus and associated complications. Soft Sci. 2024;4(2) https://doi.org/10.20517/ss.2024.02.

12. Pour SRS, Calabria D, Emamiamin A, Lazzarini E, Pace A, Guardigli M, et al. Electrochemical vs optical biosensors for point-of-care applications: a critical review. Chemosensors. 2023;11(10):546.

13. Harun-Or-Rashid M, Aktar MN, Preda V, Nasiri N. Advances in electrochemical sensors for real-time glucose monitoring. Sens Diagn. 2024;3(6):893–913.

14. Wibowo NA, Kurniawan C, Kusumahastuti DK, Setiawan A, Suharyadi E. Potential of tunneling-magnetoresistance coupled to iron-oxide nanoparticles as a novel transducer for biosensors-on-chip. J Electrochem Soc. 2024;171(1):017512.

15. Bocu R. Integration of electrochemical biosensors into modern IoT and wearable devices: an extended review. Biosensors. 2024;14(5):214.

16. Iftikhar A, Ishtiaq Q, Uzair M, Nazir QA, Ch AS, Khan ZA. Novel biomarkers in early detection of chronic kidney disease: current evidence and future directions. Indus J Biosci Res. 2025;3(5):58–66.

17. Mohammadpour-Haratbar A, Mohammadpour-Haratbar S, Zare Y, Rhee KY, Park SJ. Non-enzymatic electrochemical glucose biosensors using carbon-nanofiber nanocomposites: a review. Biosensors. 2022;12(11):1004.

18. Lin J, Chen Y, Liu X, Jiang H, Wang X. Engineered intelligent electrochemical biosensors for portable point-of-care diagnostics. Chemosensors. 2025;13(4):146.

19. Rupwate D, Balachander G (2025) Advances in biosensors for early and rare disease detection: a fabrication perspective

20. Krauss TF, Miller L, Wälti C, Johnson S. Photonic and electrochemical biosensors for near-patient tests: a critical comparison. Optica. 2024;11(10):1408–18.

21. Zhang H, Zhou X, Li X, Gong P, Zhang Y, Zhao Y. Recent advancements of LSPR fiber-optic biosensing: combination methods, structure, and prospects. Biosensors. 2023;13(3):405.

22. Hao Z, Kong L, Ruan L, Deng Z. Recent advances in DNA origami-enabled optical biosensors for multi-scenario application. Nanomaterials. 2024;14(23):1968.

23. Shrikrishna NS, Sharma R, Sahoo J, Kaushik A, Gandhi S. Navigating the landscape of optical biosensors. Chem Eng J. 2024;490:151661.

24. Jarnda KV, Dai H, Ali A, Bestman PL, Trafialek J, Roberts-Jarnda GP, et al. Optical biosensors for monitoring uric acid and blood glucose using portable POCT devices: status, challenges, and future horizons. Biosensors. 2025;15(4):222.

25. Lu S, Dai Z, Cui Y, Kong DM. Development of advanced fluorescent molecular probes for organelle-targeted cell imaging. Biosensors. 2023;13(3):360.

26. Lv J, Wang J, Yang L, Liu W, Fu H, Chu PK, Liu C. Optical fiber biosensors based on surface plasmon resonance: sensing principles, structures, and prospects. Sens Diagn. 2024;3(9):1369–91.

27. Xie Y, Hou Y, Hu M, Chen H, Wang H, Zhao L, Xu J. Dual monitoring of blood acetyl-cholinesterase content and catalytic activity utilizing fluorometry-integrated surface plasmon resonance. Biosensors. 2025;15(2):118.

28. Kabashin AV, Kravets VG, Grigorenko AN. Label-free optical biosensing: going beyond the limits. Chem Soc Rev. 2023;52(18):6554–85.

29. Singh AK, Anwar M, Pradhan R, Ashar MS, Rai N, Dey S. Surface plasmon resonance-based optical biosensor: emerging diagnostic tool for early disease detection. J Biophotonics. 2023;16(7):e202200380.

30. Tselikov GI, Danilov A, Shipunova VO, Deyev SM, Kabashin AV, Grigorenko AN. Topological darkness: design of metamaterials for optical biosensing with ultrahigh sensitivity. ACS Nano. 2023;17(19):19338–48.

31. Yan T, Guo C, Wang C, Zhu K. Optical biosensing systems for biological living bodies. View. 2023;4(4):20220059.

32. Xu Y, Zhang J, Ray WZ, MacEwan MR. Implantable and semi-implantable biosensors for minimally invasive disease diagnosis. Processes. 2024;12(7):1535.

33. Sangeetha P, Ayyanar N, Prabhakar G, Rajaram S. Optical biosensors based on 2D materials: a study review. Plasmonics. 2025:1–15.

34. Bliah O, Hegde C, Tan JMR, Magdassi S. Fabrication of soft robotics by additive manufacturing: from materials to applications. Chem Rev. 2025;125(16):7275–320.

35. Duy Mac K, Su J. Optical biosensors for diagnosing neurodegenerative diseases. NPJ Biosens. 2025;2(1):20.

36. Randviir EP, Banks CE. Review of electrochemical impedance spectroscopy for bioanalytical sensors. Anal Methods. 2022;14(45):4602–24.

37. Štukovnik Z, Bren U. Recent developments in electrochemical-impedimetric biosensors for virus detection. Int J Mol Sci. 2022;23(24):15922.

38. Arman S, Tilley RD, Gooding JJ. Electrochemical impedance as a tool for examining cell biology and subcellular mechanisms: merits, limits, and future prospects. Analyst. 2024;149(2):269–89.

39. Ribeiro JA, Jorge PA. Applications of electrochemical impedance spectroscopy in disease diagnosis: a review. Sens Actuators Rep. 2024;8:100205.

40. Lazanas AC, Prodromidis MI. Electrochemical impedance spectroscopy—a tutorial. ACS Meas Sci Au. 2023;3(3):162–93.

41. Chen YS, Huang CH, Pai PC, Seo J, Lei KF. Microfluidics-based impedance biosensors: a review. Biosensors. 2023;13(1):83.

42. Akhtarian S, Kaur Brar S, Rezai P. Electrochemical impedance spectroscopy-based microfluidic biosensor using cell-imprinted polymers for bacteria detection. Biosensors. 2024;14(9):445.

43. Radhakrishnan S, Mathew M, Rout CS. Microfluidic sensors based on two-dimensional materials for chemical and biological assessments. Mater Adv. 2022;3(4):1874–904.

44. Magar HS, Hassan RY, Mulchandani A. Electrochemical impedance spectroscopy (EIS): principles, construction, and biosensing applications. Sensors (Basel). 2021;21(19):6578.

45. Ribeiro LV, Cancino-Bernardi J, Razzino CDA, Machado TR, Tuesta MA, Zucolotto V. Electrochemical impedance spectroscopy for early diagnosis of mycobacterium tuberculosis using CFP10:ESAT6 protein detection. Front Sens. 2024;5:1512936.

46. de Amorim RS, Serrano PA, Nunes GE, Bechtold IH. Improving accuracy and reliability of an electrochemical impedance spectroscopy aptamer-based biosensor. Results Chem. 2024;7:101488.

47. Sekhon S, et al. Capacitive sensors for label-free detection in high-ionic-strength environments: a review of EIS biosensors. Biosensors. 2024;15:491.

48. Narita F, Wang Z, Kurita H, Li Z, Shi Y, Jia Y, Soutis C. Piezoelectric and magnetostrictive biosensor materials for detection of COVID-19 and other viruses: a review. Adv Mater. 2021;33(1):2005448.

49. Gouda M, Ghazzawy HS, Alqahtani N, Li X. Acoustic sensors as chemical detecting tools for biological cells and bioactivities. Molecules. 2023;28(12):4855.

50. Qureshi S, Hanif M, Jeoti V, Stojanović GM, Khan MT. Fabrication of SAW sensors on flexible substrates: challenges and future. Results Eng. 2024;22:102323.

51. Aleixandre M, Horrillo MC. Recent advances in SAW sensors for detection of cancer biomarkers. Biosensors. 2025;15(2):88.

52. Subhan MA, Neogi N, Choudhury KP, Rahman MM. Metal/metal-oxide nanoscale materials in biosensor applications: recent advances. Chem. 2025;13(2):49.

53. Mujahid A, Afzal A, Dickert FL. High-frequency acoustic sensors—QCMs, SAWs, and FBARs: chemical and biochemical applications. Sensors (Basel). 2019;19(20):4395.
54. Gouda MM. Recent trends in acoustic sensor applications. Sound Vib. 2025;59(2):3188.
55. Pohanka M. Piezoelectric chemosensors and biosensors in medical diagnostics. Biosensors. 2025;15(3):197.
56. Saleh S, Alkalamouni H, Antar K, Rahme J, Kazan M, Karam P, et al. Quartz crystal microbalance-based biosensor for rapid and ultrasensitive SARS-CoV-2 detection. J Pharm Biomed Anal Open. 2025;5:100071.
57. Alanazi N, Almutairi M, Alodhayb AN. Quartz crystal microbalance for chemical and biological sensing applications: a review. Sens Imaging. 2023;24(1):10.
58. Ntimtsas A, Gizeli E. Portable surface acoustic wave platform coupled with paper-based capillary fluidics for real-time biosensing. Sens Actuators A Phys. 2024;378:115814.
59. Chen Q, Yao Y, Ao J, Yu X, Wu D, Shou M, et al. Advances in quartz crystal microbalance relative humidity sensors: a review. Measurement. 2024:116415.
60. Ba Hashwan SS, Khir MHM, Nawi IM, Ahmad MR, Hanif M, Zahoor F, et al. Piezoelectric MEMS sensors and actuators for gas detection applications: a review. Discov Nano. 2023;18(1):25.
61. Hao R, Liu L, Yuan J, Wu L, Lei S. Field effect transistor biosensors: design strategies and sensitive assay applications. Biosensors. 2023;13(4):426.
62. Zou J, Bai H, Zhang L, Shen Y, Yang C, Zhuang W, et al. Ion-sensitive field effect transistor biosensors for biomarker detection: progress and challenges. J Mater Chem B. 2024;12(35):8523–42.
63. Ghasemi F, Salimi A. 2D-based field effect transistors as biosensing platforms: principles and biomedical applications. Microchem J. 2023;187:108432.
64. Yang W, Feng W, Hou S, Hao Z, Huang C, Pan Y. Development of GFETs for biometric applications. Sens Diagn. 2025;
65. Li H, Li D, Chen H, Yue X, Fan K, Dong L, Wang G. Silicon nanowire field effect transistor biosensor with high sensitivity. Sensors (Basel). 2023;23(15):6808.
66. Sengupta J, Hussain CM. Carbon nanotube-based field effect transistor biosensors for biomedical applications: decadal developments and advancements (2016–2025). Biosensors. 2025;15(5):296.
67. Sakata T. Signal transduction interfaces for field-effect transistor-based biosensors. Commun Chem. 2024;7(1):35.
68. Nguyen TTH, Nguyen CM, Huynh MA, Vu HH, Nguyen TK, Nguyen NT. Field effect transistor-based wearable biosensors for healthcare monitoring. J Nanobiotechnology. 2023;21(1):411.
69. Chen S, Sun Y, Fan X, Xu Y, Chen S, Zhang X, et al. Two-dimensional material-based field-effect transistor biosensors: accomplishments, mechanisms, and perspectives. J Nanobiotechnol. 2023;21(1):144.
70. Janićijević Z, Baraban L. Integration strategies and formats in field-effect transistor chemo- and biosensors: a critical review. ACS Sens. 2025;10(4):2431–52.
71. Sun M, Wang S, Liang Y, Wang C, Zhang Y, Liu H, et al. Flexible graphene field-effect transistors and their application in biomedical sensing. Nano Micro Lett. 2025;17(1):34.
72. Kim HE, Schuck A, Park H, Chung DR, Kang M, Kim YS. Dual-mode graphene field-effect transistor biosensor with isothermal nucleic acid amplification. Biosensors. 2024;14(2):91.
73. Novodchuk I, Bajcsy M, Yavuz M. Graphene-based field effect transistor biosensors for breast-cancer detection: a review. Carbon. 2021;172:431–53.
74. Rai H, Singh KR, Natarajan A, Pandey SS. Field effect transistor-based electronic devices integrated with CMOS technology for biosensing. Talanta Open. 2024:100394.
75. Chao L, Liang Y, Hu X. Field effect transistor biosensors for drug screening applications: recent advances. Analyst. 2025;

76. Jang M, Na W, Lee M, Jung S, Woo Y, Yoo HY, et al. Light-induced field effect transistor-based biosensor using aptamer and ReS$_2$ single-crystal layer for exosome detection. Mater Today Bio. 2025:102281.

77. Rani AQ, Zhu B, Ueda H, Kitaguchi T. Homogeneous immunosensors based on fluorescence or bioluminescence using antibody engineering: recent progress. Analyst. 2023;148(7):1422–9.

78. Tyśkiewicz R, Fedorowicz M, Nakonieczna A, Zielińska P, Kwiatek M, Mizak L. Electrochemical, optical, and mass-based immunosensors: comprehensive review of bacillus anthracis detection methods. Anal Biochem. 2023;675:115215.

79. Soni DK, Ahmad R, Dubey SK. Biosensor for detection of listeria monocytogenes: emerging trends. Crit Rev Microbiol. 2018;44(5):590–608.

80. Karachaliou CE, Koukouvinos G, Goustouridis D, Raptis I, Kakabakos S, Petrou P, Livaniou E. Cortisol immunosensors: a literature review. Biosensors. 2023;13(2):285.

81. Cancelliere R, Cosio T, Campione E, Corvino M, D'Amico MP, Micheli L, et al. Label-free electrochemical immunosensor for interleukin-6 detection in psoriasis serum samples. Front Chem. 2023;11:1251360.

82. Shen Y, Zhao S, Chen F, Lv Y, Fu L. Enhancing sensitivity and selectivity: electrochemical immunosensors for organophosphate analysis. Biosensors. 2024;14(10):496.

83. Sobhanparast S, Shahbazi-Derakhshi P, Soleymani J, Amiri-Sadeghan A, Herischi A, Chaparzadeh N, Aftabi Y. Electrochemical immunosensor based on biomaterials for carcinoembryonic antigen detection. Sci Rep. 2025;15(1):25396.

84. Li H, Pan TG, He S, Sun H, Cao X, Ye Y. Electrochemical immunosensor for rapid and sensitive detection of sesame allergens Ses i 4 and Ses i 5. Foods. 2025;14(1):115.

85. Heng W. Smart masks for in situ exhaled-breath condensate harvesting and analysis. California Inst Technol. 2025;

86. Dave S, Das J, Sillanpää M. Nanomaterials and point of care technologies. CRC Press; 2024.

87. Panahi A, Ghafar-Zadeh E. Emerging field-effect transistor biosensors for life science applications. Bioengineering. 2023;10(7):793.

88. Eswaran M, Chokkiah B, Pandit S, Rahimi S, Dhanusuraman R, Aleem M, Mijakovic I. A road map toward field-effect transistor biosensor technology for early stage cancer detection. Small Methods. 2022;6(10):2200809.

89. Vu CA, Chen WY. Field-effect transistor biosensors for biomedical applications: recent advances and future prospects. Sensors (Basel). 2019;19(19):4214.

90. Rai H, Singh KR, Natarajan A, Pandey SS. Advances in field effect transistor based electronic devices integrated with CMOS technology for biosensing. Talanta Open. 2024:100394.

91. Police Patil AV, Chuang YS, Li C, Wu CC. Recent advances in electrochemical immunosensors with nanomaterial assistance for signal amplification. Biosensors. 2023;13(1):125.

92. Janik-Karpinska E, Ceremuga M, Niemcewicz M, Podogrocki M, Stela M, Cichon N, Bijak M. Immunosensors—the future of pathogen real-time detection. Sensors (Basel). 2022;22(24):9757.

93. Hadžić S, Trkulja A, Alihodžić I. Immunosensors: recent advances and applications. In: Proc Int Conf med biol Eng. Cham: Springer Int Publ; 2021. p. 138–51.

94. Aydin M, Aydin EB, Sezgintürk MK. Advances in immunosensor technology. In: Adv Clin Chem, vol. 102; 2021. p. 1–62.

95. Karachaliou CE, Koukouvinos G, Goustouridis D, Raptis I, Kakabakos S, Livaniou E, Petrou P. Recent developments in the field of optical immunosensors focusing on a label-free, white light reflectance spectroscopy-based immunosensing platform. Sensors. 2022;22(14):5114.

96. Rosa BG, Akingbade OE, Guo X, Gonzalez-Macia L, Crone MA, Cameron LP, et al. Multiplexed immunosensors for point-of-care diagnostic applications. Biosens Bioelectron. 2022;203:114050.

97. O'Brien C, Khor CK, Ardalan S, Ignaszak A. Multiplex electrochemical sensing platforms for the detection of breast cancer biomarkers. Front Med Technol. 2024;6:1360510.

98. Vo DK, Trinh KTL. Advances in wearable biosensors for healthcare: current trends, applications, and future perspectives. Biosensors. 2024;14(11):560.
99. Ghazizadeh E, Naseri Z, Deigner HP, Rahimi H, Altintas Z. Approaches of wearable and implantable biosensor towards developing precision medicine. Front Med. 2024;11:1390634.
100. Mathew M, Radhakrishnan S, Vaidyanathan A, Chakraborty B, Rout CS. Flexible and wearable electrochemical biosensors based on two-dimensional materials: recent developments. Anal Bioanal Chem. 2021;413(3):727–62.
101. Sadighbayan D, Hasanzadeh M, Ghafar-Zadeh E. Biosensing based on field-effect transistors (FET): recent progress and challenges. TrAC Trends Anal Chem. 2020;133:116067.
102. Singh R, Gupta R, Bansal D, Bhateria R, Sharma M. A review on recent trends and future developments in electrochemical sensing. ACS Omega. 2024;9(7):7336–56.
103. Halima HB, Errachid A, Jaffrezic-Renault N. The future of commercializing FET-based biosensors. In: Field-Effect transistor biosensors for rapid pathogen detection. Elsevier; 2024. p. 195–223.
104. Mehta D, Gupta D, Kafle A, Kaur S, Nagaiah TC. Advances and challenges in nanomaterial-based electrochemical immunosensors for small cell lung cancer biomarker neuron-specific enolase. ACS Omega. 2023;9(1):33–51.
105. Nguyen TTH, Nguyen CM, Huynh MA, Vu HH, Nguyen TK, Nguyen NT. Field effect transistor-based wearable biosensors for healthcare monitoring. J Nanobiotechnol. 2023;21(1):411.
106. Jones A, Dhanapala L, Kankanamage RN, Kumar CV, Rusling JF. Multiplexed immunosensors and immunoarrays. Anal Chem. 2019;92(1):345–62.
107. Liao Z, Wang J, Zhang P, Zhang Y, Miao Y, Gao S, et al. Recent advances in microfluidic chip-integrated electronic biosensors for multiplexed detection. Biosens Bioelectron. 2018;121:272–80.
108. Askarzadeh N, Mehrizi AA, Mohammadi J, Rabbani H, Ghourchian H, Mottaghitalab F. A review of biomaterials for developing high-performance immunosensors: rigid and flexible platforms. TrAC Trends Anal Chem. 2025:118343.
109. Aizawa M. Immunosensors. In: Biosensor principles and applications. Elsevier; 2019. p. 249–66.
110. Morawska K, Sikora T, Grabka M, Wiśnik-Sawka M, Witkiewicz Z. Early detection of threat agents: a review of bioimmunosensors and their prospects. Crit Rev Anal Chem. 2025:1–15.

Chapter 3
Applications and Future Trends

This chapter focuses on the biomedical role of biosensors, tracing their evolution from diagnostic tools to intelligent health-monitoring systems. Section 3.1 outlines key clinical applications, including disease detection, cancer biomarker monitoring, therapeutic drug tracking, and wearable health technologies that enable continuous patient observation. Section 3.2 discusses emerging directions, miniaturization, smartphone-linked devices, nanomaterial-enhanced sensitivity, and AI-driven data analysis, while addressing challenges of biocompatibility, long-term performance, and ethics. Together, these sections present biosensors as integral components of modern medicine, transforming biological signals into actionable medical insight.

3.1   Biomedical Applications of Biosensors

Biosensors are increasingly vital to medical science, offering rapid and precise methods for measuring biological and chemical changes in the human body. By coupling a biological recognition element with a physical transducer, these devices convert biochemical reactions into measurable signals [1]. In biomedicine, they are used to diagnose disease, monitor treatment progress, and support preventive and personalized healthcare. Their continuous evolution, driven by nanotechnology, data analytics, and microelectronics, has transformed how clinicians and researchers gather and interpret physiological data.

3.1.1   Diagnostic Applications

The earliest practical biomedical biosensor was developed for glucose monitoring, which remains the most successful example of biosensor implementation in healthcare. The concept originated with Leland C. Clark Jr.'s oxygen electrode (1956),

A. Badnjević, L. Spahić, *Biosensors*, Series in BioEngineering,
https://doi.org/10.1007/978-3-032-15757-7_3

which was later modified with glucose oxidase to detect blood sugar [2]. This invention laid the foundation for the portable glucometers and continuous glucose monitoring (CGM) devices now used worldwide.

Beyond diabetes management, biosensors have become indispensable for infectious disease diagnostics. Electrochemical and optical immunosensors are used to identify antigens or antibodies associated with diseases such as HIV, hepatitis B and C, malaria, and SARS-CoV-2. During the COVID-19 pandemic, portable CRISPR-Cas and electrochemical biosensors enabled rapid, accurate detection of viral RNA, demonstrating the potential for decentralized point-of-care testing (Table 3.1).

These devices offer distinct advantages over conventional laboratory assays: faster turnaround, reduced reagent consumption, and the ability to test at the bedside or in remote areas.

3.1.2   Cancer and Molecular Diagnostics

In **oncology,** biosensors are being developed to detect tumor biomarkers long before clinical symptoms appear. SPR and fluorescence-based optical sensors can measure trace levels of molecules such as prostate-specific antigen (PSA), carcinoembryonic antigen (CEA), or HER2 [3]. The ability to monitor these markers in real time has improved early diagnosis and personalized therapy selection.

Table 3.1 Comparison of biosensor-based and conventional diagnostic methods

Diagnostic Method	Detection Principle	Typical Analysis Time	Sensitivity (Detection Limit)	Portability	Cost per Test	Example Application
ELISA (enzyme-linked immunosorbent assay)	Enzyme–substrate colorimetric reaction	2–4 h	~ng/mL	Low	Moderate	Detection of viral antigens
PCR (polymerase chain reaction)	DNA amplification and fluorescence	2–6 h	~fg/mL (DNA level)	Low	High	SARS-CoV-2, genetic testing
Electrochemical biosensor	Current or voltage change upon biomolecular binding	5–20 min	~pg/mL	High	Low	Glucose, cholesterol, lactate
Optical biosensor (SPR/ fluorescence)	Change in refractive index or fluorescence	10–30 min	~pg/mL	Moderate	Moderate–high	Protein–protein interactions
Paper-based biosensor (CRISPR-based)	Visual signal via lateral flow or fluorescence	15–45 min	~pg/mL	Very high	Very low	Rapid viral RNA detection

DNA and RNA biosensors (genosensors) extend these capabilities to molecular diagnostics. By recognizing specific nucleotide sequences, they can identify mutations linked to hereditary cancers, viral infections, or antimicrobial resistance [4]. Their high specificity and rapid response make them attractive alternatives to polymerase chain reaction (PCR) testing, especially for field or bedside use (Table 3.2).

3.1.3 Therapeutic and Drug-Monitoring Applications

Biosensors are also used to monitor therapeutic drug levels in biological fluids, ensuring that concentrations remain within a safe and effective range. In chemotherapy, for example, drug levels can vary significantly among patients; biosensor-based therapeutic drug monitoring (TDM) helps minimize toxicity and enhance efficacy. Electrochemical biosensors can detect drugs such as theophylline, phenytoin, or antibiotics directly from blood or saliva samples. More advanced systems use aptamers, synthetic oligonucleotides that bind drugs with high specificity, to improve selectivity and reproducibility [5]. Implantable biosensors represent the next stage of therapeutic monitoring. These devices can measure glucose, lactate, or oxygen directly in tissues and communicate with external pumps to automatically adjust drug delivery. This principle underlies the development of closed-loop insulin delivery systems, often described as "artificial pancreas" technology (Table 3.3).

3.1.4 Physiological and Wearable Monitoring

The miniaturization of biosensors has enabled continuous health tracking through wearable and skin-mounted devices. Flexible biosensors can monitor heart rate, oxygen saturation, sweat composition, hydration level, and other physiological parameters. Electrochemical sensors embedded in wristbands or adhesive patches

Table 3.2 Common cancer biomarkers detected by biosensors

Biomarker	Associated Cancer	Biosensor Type	Biorecognition Element	Detection Limit	Sample Type
PSA (prostate-specific antigen)	Prostate cancer	Electrochemical / SPR	Antibody	0.1 ng/mL	Serum
CEA (carcinoembryonic antigen)	Colorectal, lung, breast	Optical (fluorescence)	Antibody	0.05 ng/mL	Plasma
HER2 (human epidermal growth factor receptor 2)	Breast cancer	SPR / electrochemical	Antibody or aptamer	0.01 ng/mL	Serum
CA-125 (cancer antigen 125)	Ovarian cancer	Electrochemical	Antibody	0.5 U/mL	Serum
MicroRNA-21	Multiple cancers	DNA biosensor	ssDNA probe	10 fM	Serum, saliva

Table 3.3 Examples of biosensors used in therapeutic monitoring

Target Drug	Biosensor Type	Recognition Element	Transduction Mechanism	Detection Range	Clinical Purpose
Theophylline	Electrochemical	Aptamer	Current change (CV)	$0.1\text{--}100\ \mu M$	Asthma and COPD control
Phenytoin	Optical (SPR)	Antibody	Refractive index shift	$0.5\text{--}50\ \mu M$	Anti-epileptic drug monitoring
Methotrexate	Electrochemical	Enzyme-linked	Amperometric signal	$0.01\text{--}10\ \mu M$	Chemotherapy dosage control
Gentamicin	Piezoelectric	Aptamer	Frequency shift	$0.1\text{--}50\ \mu M$	Antibiotic therapy optimization
Cyclosporine A	Electrochemical	Antibody	Potentiometric response	$1\text{--}100\ \text{ng/mL}$	Immunosuppressive therapy tracking

detect biomarkers such as glucose, cortisol, and lactate in sweat. Optical sensors, integrated into smartwatches, measure heart rate and oxygenation using photoplethysmography (PPG). Wireless transmission of these data to smartphones or cloud systems supports personalized health management and remote medical supervision [6]. In neurological and cardiac medicine, biosensors are integrated with EEG and ECG systems for continuous monitoring. They assist in detecting arrhythmias, epilepsy episodes, or sleep irregularities (Fig. 3.1).

3.1.5 Biosensors in Critical and Preventive Medicine

In critical care settings, biosensors provide immediate information on blood gases, electrolytes, and metabolites from minimal sample volumes. Bedside sensors reduce the time between measurement and intervention—an essential factor in emergency medicine [7]. Preventive medicine also benefits from biosensor development. Devices capable of detecting early inflammatory or metabolic shifts may identify disease risks before symptoms manifest. For example, point-of-care biosensors for C-reactive protein (CRP) can signal infection or chronic inflammation, prompting early treatment (Fig. 3.2).

3.1.6 Emerging Technologies

Nanomaterials and AI are redefining the scope of biomedical biosensors. Nanostructured electrodes increase surface area and sensitivity, enabling the detection of picomolar concentrations of analytes. Graphene, gold nanoparticles, and

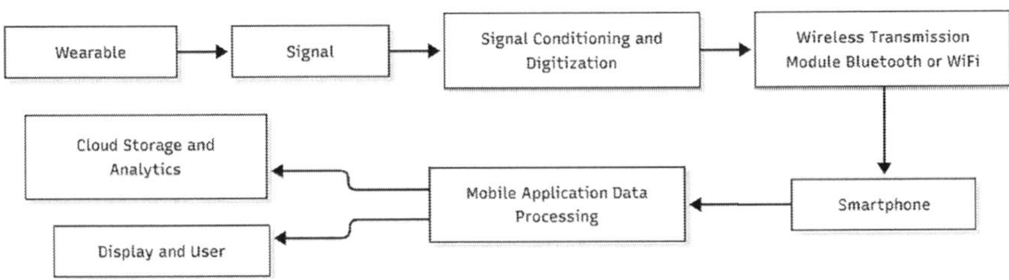

Fig. 3.1 Flowchart of data transmission from wearable biosensor to smartphone application

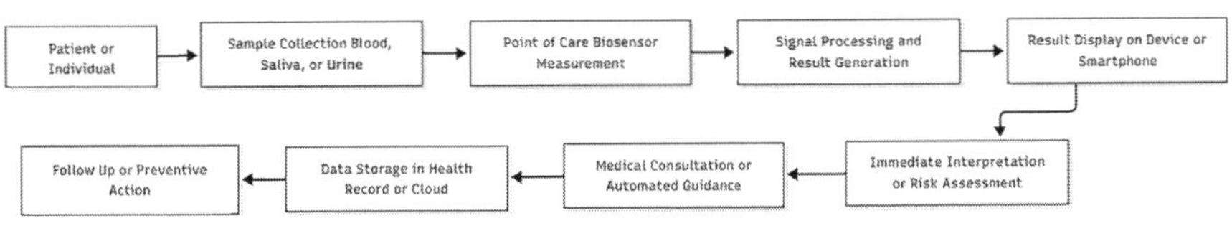

Fig. 3.2 Workflow for preventive screening using point-of-care biosensors

carbon nanotubes are particularly promising for next-generation biosensors. Meanwhile, AI and ML algorithms enhance biosensor signal processing, noise reduction, and pattern recognition. These tools enable predictive analytics, for instance, forecasting glucose fluctuations or detecting early signs of cardiac stress based on signal trends [8]. Integration with the Internet of Things (IoT) now allows biosensors to communicate with healthcare networks, supporting telemedicine and population-scale health monitoring.

3.2   Future Trends and Challenges in Biosensors

The use of biosensors in healthcare and medicine has grown rapidly in recent years, reflecting their versatility and clinical value. These devices are now essential tools for disease diagnosis, patient monitoring, and personalized health management. Their precision and adaptability have also driven their expansion into other fields, including agriculture, food safety, environmental analysis, and biotechnology.

Biosensors provide deep mechanistic insight into biological systems at the molecular level. As analytical instruments, they enable the detection of a wide range of substances, from simple ions such as calcium (Ca^{2+}) to complex biomolecules like enzymes, antibodies, and nucleic acids. This capacity has made biosensors indispensable across disciplines such as drug discovery, microbial and viral detection, gene therapy, and industrial bioprocess monitoring [9].

Modern biosensor research focuses on making these devices smaller, smarter, and more integrated into daily life. Recent progress has centered on miniaturization, smartphone integration, and the use of nanomaterials to enhance sensitivity and signal strength. Additionally, AI has emerged as a transformative tool for biosensor data analysis, enabling real-time interpretation, improved diagnostic accuracy, and early disease detection. At the same time, important challenges remain, particularly in biocompatibility, long-term stability, and regulatory approval. As biosensors evolve from laboratory prototypes to practical, clinical-grade devices, issues such as material safety, power management, and data privacy require continued research. The following sections discuss how these technologies are advancing—from smartphone-linked biosensors and nanomaterial-based designs to AI-driven analytical systems—while also addressing key limitations that must be overcome for broader adoption.

3.2.1   Integration of Biosensors in Smartphones

The widespread use of smartphones and their powerful computational capabilities has opened new possibilities for mobile health applications, including the integration of biosensors. These devices, when connected to or embedded within smartphones, are transforming traditional diagnostics into portable, real-time, and user-friendly platforms. This combination enables individuals to monitor various health indicators remotely, laying the foundation for accessible, decentralized healthcare systems.

Smartphone-based biosensors function in several ways: the smartphone can serve as an instrumental interface, data processor, or even as the detector itself. In many designs, the phone's camera, light source, or internal sensors are used to capture analytical signals generated by biological reactions [10]. Compared with traditional laboratory instruments such as spectrophotometers and microscopes, smartphone-integrated biosensors are far more compact, affordable, and widely accessible. This portability is particularly valuable in remote or resource-limited regions, where they can provide rapid point-of-care diagnostics for healthcare, food safety, biosecurity, and environmental monitoring.

Modern smartphones possess advanced features, high-resolution cameras, internal memory, fast processors, and sophisticated operating systems, that make them comparable to small computers. These features enable them to support biosensing operations that once required skilled technicians and complex laboratory equipment. For example, smartphone-based diagnostic kits can detect infectious agents or analyze body fluids in real time, drastically reducing turnaround times for clinical decisions. Several approaches have been explored to fully integrate biosensors into smartphones. The ideal configuration is a fully autonomous biosensor in which the biorecognition element and the transducer are seamlessly integrated with the smartphone detector. However, this complete integration remains challenging due to design constraints and compatibility issues. More commonly, smartphones are employed as external readout units or instrumental interfaces that connect to biosensing modules via wired or wireless communication [11]. Smartphone-based biosensors can also be applied to fluorescence-based assays, exploiting optical mechanisms such as fluorescence, chemiluminescence, or quantum dot emission. A particularly promising approach uses Förster Resonance Energy Transfer (FRET), which detects changes in fluorescence quenching between donor-acceptor molecular pairs. FRET-based smartphone biosensors can conduct single-step assays directly in liquid samples, eliminating the need for complex washing or mixing steps. This makes them ideal for fast and cost-effective diagnostic applications.

3.2.2 Types of Smartphone-Based Biosensors

Smartphone-based biosensors can be classified according to their detection mechanism and transduction method. The most common types are optical, SPR, and electrochemical biosensors [12]. Each category utilizes distinct principles to detect and quantify biological or chemical analytes, but all share the advantage of portability, affordability, and direct data visualization through the smartphone interface.

Optical biosensors integrated with smartphones are among the most established and versatile formats. They leverage smartphones' high-resolution cameras and advanced imaging software to detect optical signals from biological interactions. The earliest applications involved attaching miniature optical accessories to smartphones to create compact microscopes capable of visualizing blood cells, microorganisms, and other biological samples [13]. Recent innovations have enabled the detection of nucleic acids, viruses, nanoparticles, and proteins using miniaturized optical components and advanced image analysis algorithms. Improvements in sensor resolution and camera sensitivity now allow these systems to achieve nanoscale imaging, once possible only with laboratory-grade equipment. By using fluorescent dyes, colorimetric reactions, or quantum dots as labels, smartphone optical biosensors can convert biological reactions into visible color changes or luminescent signals that are instantly analyzed through mobile applications.

SPR mobile phone biosensors rely on refractometric sensing, a technique that measures how light interacts with the surface of a thin metallic layer, typically gold. When a biological interaction occurs on the sensor surface, such as antigen-antibody binding, the refractive index changes, leading to a measurable shift in the SPR signal. In smartphone-based SPR biosensors, compact optical assemblies are connected to the smartphone's camera or light source to detect these shifts. The smartphone acts as both the signal processor and display interface, providing immediate feedback. This approach enables portable, label-free detection of biomolecules and has been used in applications such as food safety testing, disease biomarker detection, and environmental monitoring.

Electrochemical biosensors adapted for smartphones are gaining popularity because of their simplicity, low cost, and quantitative capabilities. They measure electrical changes—such as current, voltage, or impedance—produced by biochemical reactions on the electrode surface. These devices can detect important biological molecules, including proteins, nucleic acids, metabolites, and metal ions, making them useful in clinical diagnostics, pollution control, and food safety analysis [14]. In typical configurations, the smartphone communicates with the electrochemical sensor via a wireless module (Bluetooth, NFC, or Wi-Fi) or a wired interface through the phone's charging port. The smartphone app records and interprets the electrochemical data, converting it into readable results for the user. This method makes advanced quantitative testing accessible without the need for large benchtop analyzers.

3.2.3 Miniaturization of Biosensors

The trend toward miniaturizing biosensors has reshaped how biomedical analysis, environmental monitoring, and food safety evaluation are conducted. Compact and portable designs have made biosensors faster, more efficient, and easier to use in real-world settings. Miniaturization enables these devices to perform highly sensitive, selective analyses at the point of care, eliminating the need for large, expensive laboratory instruments.

Recent technological advances have produced **microfluidic-based biosensors** and handheld diagnostic systems that perform complex biochemical analyses with only a few microliters of sample. These platforms integrate multiple analytical steps, such as sample collection, reagent mixing, reaction processing, and signal detection, into a single, miniature chip [15]. Microfluidic biosensors are often described as "labs on a chip," since they replicate the functionality of an entire laboratory within a palm-sized device. Portable biosensors have already been adapted for everyday measurements such as temperature, pH, and blood glucose. However, researchers continue to face challenges in designing small-scale systems that can achieve high accuracy without relying on external laboratory instruments. Innovations in microfabrication, microelectromechanical systems (MEMS), and integrated electronics are helping overcome these limitations by enabling higher precision in smaller formats. Miniaturized biosensors for POC testing are typically built to be low-cost, rapid, and highly selective. They use simplified signaling techniques to minimize the need for bulky optical components or high-power sources. These characteristics make them ideal for use in low-resource or remote locations, where access to laboratory infrastructure is limited. For instance, portable biosensors are being used to detect infectious diseases, analyze food contaminants, and monitor environmental pollutants directly in the field.

The miniaturization of biosensors has been heavily influenced by advancements in the microelectronics industry, particularly the scaling principle that has continually reduced transistor size while increasing computational power. This concept has inspired similar downsizing in biosensor design, from millimeter-scale systems to microscale and nanoscale devices.

Shrinking biosensors to the microscale offers several advantages. It reduces sample and reagent consumption, improves reaction kinetics, and increases surface-to-volume ratios, enhancing signal strength and detection sensitivity. However, two primary processes must be optimized: reaction-transport kinetics and signal transduction efficiency [16]. Reaction-transport kinetics describe how quickly target molecules reach the sensor surface, while signal transduction efficiency determines how effectively these interactions are converted into measurable outputs. Achieving a balance between these processes ensures faster response times and lower detection limits. As biosensors become smaller and more efficient, they are increasingly integrated into wearable and implantable systems for continuous health monitoring. These developments mark a major step toward the realization of fully autonomous diagnostic devices capable of operating directly within or on the human body.

Nanomaterials have revolutionized biosensor technology by dramatically improving detection sensitivity, selectivity, and response time. Defined by dimensions on the nanometer scale, these materials occupy the space between bulk matter and single atoms, giving them unique electrical, optical, and chemical properties that can be precisely engineered for biosensing applications. The use of nanomaterials in biosensors has expanded rapidly because their high surface-to-volume ratio allows for greater immobilization of biorecognition molecules on the sensor surface. This increased surface area increases the number of active binding sites for target analytes, resulting in stronger, more reliable signals. When incorporated into electrode-based or optical systems, nanomaterials significantly amplify the signal-to-noise ratio, enabling the detection of extremely low concentrations of biomolecules.

Common nanomaterials used in biosensing include gold nanoparticles, graphene, carbon nanotubes, quantum dots, and metal oxides. Each type provides distinct advantages. Gold nanoparticles, for example, are biocompatible and excellent conductors, making them ideal for electrochemical sensors. Graphene and carbon nanotubes offer outstanding electrical conductivity and mechanical flexibility, which are valuable for the development of wearable biosensors [17]. Quantum dots, on the other hand, possess unique photoluminescent properties that are useful for fluorescent or optical detection. Recent advancements have focused on tailoring the structure, size, and chemical composition of nanomaterials to further enhance biosensor performance. Researchers are developing biomimetic optical nanomaterials and bio-inspired mechanically adaptive materials that improve both selectivity and signal precision. These engineered materials not only amplify detection signals but also enhance biocompatibility and stability, enabling biosensors to function reliably over longer periods.

Nanomaterial-based biosensors have become essential for real-time detection of disease biomarkers, offering tremendous potential in early diagnosis and therapeutic monitoring. For instance, sensors built with nanostructured electrodes can detect cancer-associated proteins, pathogens, and toxins with remarkable accuracy. Their high reproducibility and compact design make them suitable for both clinical and environmental applications. Furthermore, luminescent nanomaterials doped with rare-earth elements, such as yttrium oxide (Y_2O_3) doped with erbium or ytterbium, are emerging as promising tools for bioimaging. These materials emit visible light via anti-Stokes emission when excited by near-infrared radiation, enabling safe, non-invasive medical imaging [18].

In tissue engineering, nanoparticle-reinforced polymeric composites are being used to create materials that are both biodegradable and mechanically robust. Carbon nanotubes, graphene nanoribbons, and hydroxyapatite nanoparticles, for example, improve the structural strength of biopolymers used in bone regeneration. The high surface area and chemical reactivity of these materials enhance cross-linking within the polymer matrix, resulting in better mechanical stability and controlled degradation.

Despite their benefits, the use of nanomaterials introduces challenges in biocompatibility and in immobilization techniques. Achieving stable and uniform binding of biological molecules to nanomaterial surfaces is critical. Functionalization—either by adding chemical groups directly during synthesis or by applying specialized polymer coatings—ensures consistent attachment and reduces toxicity. Carbon-based nanomaterials such as graphene quantum dots have shown great promise due to their chemical stability, tunable fluorescence, and low toxicity. These have even been used to build electrochemical sensors capable of detecting neurotransmitters like epinephrine at nanomolar levels with minimal interference from other biological compounds.

3.2.4   Artificial Intelligence in Biosensor Data Analysis

The incorporation of AI into biosensor technology is transforming how biological data are processed, interpreted, and applied. As biosensors become more advanced and capable of generating vast amounts of data, AI, particularly machine ML and deep learning (DL) algorithms, provides the computational power necessary to analyze complex datasets with unprecedented accuracy and speed [19].

AI-driven biosensors can identify subtle variations in biological signals that traditional analytical methods might overlook. These systems are capable of filtering noise, compensating for environmental fluctuations, and recognizing non-linear relationships among physiological variables. As a result, AI significantly enhances biosensor sensitivity, precision, and diagnostic reliability, enabling more personalized and predictive healthcare.

AI offers a range of benefits that improve both the performance and the usability of biosensors [20]:

- Advanced data management: AI algorithms can efficiently handle massive, high-dimensional datasets collected from multiple sensors, ensuring that meaningful information is extracted from noisy or incomplete data.
- Pattern Recognition and Anomaly Detection: Through supervised and unsupervised learning, AI can detect minute patterns or anomalies within biosensor readings—critical for identifying early signs of diseases or environmental changes.
- Real-time monitoring and feedback: ML enables biosensors to process data in real time, providing instant alerts or adaptive responses when abnormal readings occur, such as glucose spikes or cardiac irregularities.
- Early disease diagnosis: AI systems can detect early biomarkers of disease long before symptoms appear, supporting preventive healthcare and early interventions.
- Personalized medicine: By integrating patient-specific data, AI can help tailor treatment regimens, monitor therapy effectiveness, and recommend adjustments based on individual responses.

AI-enhanced biosensors have applications extending well beyond healthcare. In medicine, wearable AI-enabled biosensors continuously monitor glucose levels, heart rate, oxygen saturation, or stress-related biochemical markers. In environmental monitoring, they help detect pollutants, toxins, and pathogens in real time, while in food safety, AI helps track spoilage indicators and contaminants. In clinical diagnostics, integrating AI enables biosensors to move beyond static measurements toward dynamic predictive models, improving clinical decision-making. For example, in diabetes management, AI-based glucose sensors can predict hypoglycemic events by analyzing real-time glucose trends, allowing automated insulin adjustments.

The rapid progress of AI in biosensing is closely linked to advances in computing hardware. Deep learning models require extensive parallel processing, often achieved using graphics processing units (GPUs) or tensor processing units (TPUs)

These specialized chips enable the efficient training of neural networks on massive datasets. Reinforcement learning has also contributed to optimizing computation processes, such as faster matrix multiplication used in neural model training [21]. Companies like Google have developed custom AI processors (e.g., TensorFlow's TPU architecture) that dramatically increase the efficiency of biosensor data analysis. The development of smaller, energy-efficient AI models through techniques like knowledge distillation, model pruning, and structural sparsity has made it feasible to integrate intelligent algorithms directly into portable and wearable devices. This progress allows biosensors to operate autonomously without constant cloud-based computation, reducing latency and preserving privacy. As AI systems continue to evolve, biosensors will not only collect and display data but also interpret, predict, and adapt to biological changes. This transition from data acquisition to data intelligence marks a crucial step toward creating next-generation biosensors capable of autonomous medical decision support, continuous health assessment, and early disease prevention.

3.2.5 Challenges in Biocompatibility and Long-Term Stability

Despite their remarkable progress, biosensors still face major obstacles related to biocompatibility, toxicity, and long-term stability, particularly when nanomaterials or implantable components are involved. As biosensors move from laboratory prototypes to clinical applications, ensuring their safe, reliable, and sustained operation within biological environments becomes a primary concern.

The increasing use of nanomaterials in biosensors introduces unique safety challenges. These materials, while advantageous for improving sensitivity and signal strength, can pose health risks if inhaled, ingested, or absorbed through the skin. Nanoparticles have the potential to enter biological systems and circulate through the bloodstream, where they may accumulate in organs or interact with cellular structures in harmful ways [22]. Studies have shown that carbon-based nanomaterials, for instance, can cause adverse effects on the respiratory, circulatory, and nervous systems.

Assessing nanotoxicity remains complex due to a lack of standardized testing methods to evaluate the long-term biological effects of engineered nanomaterials. Existing in vitro and in vivo studies often yield limited or inconsistent data, making it difficult to fully predict human health risks. Future research must therefore focus on developing comprehensive toxicity profiles, identifying safe concentration thresholds, and determining how nanomaterials degrade within the body over time.

A key direction in biosensor research is the development of biodegradable, implantable sensors that can monitor physiological processes directly within the body. For these devices to be viable, they must combine biocompatibility, mechanical stability, and controlled degradation. The goal is for such sensors to operate effectively over their intended lifespan and then safely dissolve without causing inflammation or immune reactions. However, several engineering challenges persist. Achieving consistent electrical and mechanical performance in biodegradable materials is difficult. Metals such as magnesium and molybdenum can be used in bioresorbable batteries, while biopolymers such as silk and cellulose have potential for flexible, degradable structures [23]. Yet both categories face limitations: metals can corrode unpredictably, and polymers may lose structural integrity too quickly in aqueous environments. Another challenge lies in power supply and energy management. Implantable sensors require compact, efficient, and long-lasting energy sources. Researchers are exploring solutions such as energy harvesting from body heat or motion, wireless power transfer, and bioresorbable microbatteries. Although promising, these technologies often struggle with maintaining output stability and efficiency under biological conditions.

Implantable sensors also encounter difficulties with data transmission inside the human body. Biological tissues can attenuate radio-frequency (RF) signals, leading to reduced communication efficiency and increased power consumption. Ensuring secure, low-power wireless connectivity is essential, especially when sensors transmit sensitive medical data. Advanced designs using inductive coupling and trust-based communication protocols in wireless body area networks (WBANs) are being explored to enhance safety and reliability.

The foreign body response remains one of the most persistent issues in long-term biosensor implantation. When sensors are placed in tissue, the immune system may recognize them as foreign objects, triggering inflammation and the formation of fibrous encapsulation. This not only isolates the sensor from surrounding tissues but also leads to signal drift, decreased sensitivity, and eventual sensor failure. Degradation products from both polymeric and metallic materials can also provoke local or systemic immune reactions. Small metallic particles may migrate to distant organs, while polymer fragments often remain near the implantation site, causing localized irritation [24]. Researchers are working to mitigate these effects through encapsulation coatings and surface modifications that improve tissue integration and control degradation rates.

Over-extended use, biosensors may experience signal drift due to material fatigue, biofouling, or changes in the sensor's microenvironment. Drift can occur in two main forms: offset drift, a gradual shift in baseline readings, and sensitivity drift, a slow loss of responsiveness. These issues compromise data accuracy and reliability, particularly for implantable sensors intended for continuous monitoring. To address this, modern designs incorporate auto-calibration, drift compensation algorithms, and self-healing materials that restore sensor function over time. However, achieving consistent performance in vivo remains difficult because biological environments vary in temperature, pH, and ionic composition.

Beyond technical challenges, biosensor development must address ethical and ecological factors. Safe disposal or biodegradation is critical to avoid environmental contamination from electronic waste or residual nanomaterials. In addition, as biosensors become more closely integrated with the human body, especially in wearable and implantable forms, issues of data privacy, security, and user consent become increasingly important [25]. For biosensors to achieve full clinical adoption, they must enhance patients' quality of life while remaining affordable, comfortable, and sustainable. This includes developing recyclable materials, ensuring the disposability of ingestible sensors, and minimizing user discomfort through flexible, ergonomic designs. Continued progress in material science, microfabrication, and bioengineering will be essential to overcoming these challenges and enabling the next generation of safe, long-lasting biosensors.

References

1. Vo DK, Trinh KTL. Advances in wearable biosensors for healthcare: current trends, applications, and future perspectives. Biosensors. 2024;14(11):560.
2. Hemdan M, Ali MA, Doghish AS, Mageed SSA, Elazab IM, Khalil MM, et al. Innovations in biosensor technologies for healthcare diagnostics and therapeutic drug monitoring: applications, progress, and research challenges. Sensors (Basel). 2024;24(16):5143.
3. Wasfi A, Tayfor M, Ismail A, Alharthi O, Awwad F. Advances in electrochemical biosensors for COVID-19 detection: progress, challenges, and perspectives. IEEE Sens J. 2025;
4. Kumar A, Maiti P. Sustainable biosensors based on biopolymers and green materials. Mater Adv. 2024;5(9):3563–86.
5. Li L, Wang T, Zhong Y, Li R, Deng W, Xiao X, et al. Nanomaterials for biosensing applications: a review. J Mater Chem B. 2024;12(5):1168–93.
6. Kaur B, Kumar S, Nedoma J, Martinek R, Marques C. Advancements in optical biosensing techniques: from fundamentals to future prospects. APL Photon. 2024;9(9)
7. Beltrán-Velasco AI, Clemente-Suárez VJ. Harnessing gut microbiota for biomimetic innovations in health and biotechnology. Biomimetics. 2025;10(2):73.
8. Valente B, Pinto H, Pereira TS, Campos R. Exploring biosensors' scientific production and research patterns: a bibliometric analysis. Sensors. 2024;24(10):3082.
9. Abdelfattah MA, Jamali SS, Kashaninejad N, Nguyen NT. Wearable biosensors for health monitoring: advances in graphene-based technologies. Nanoscale Horiz. 2025;10:1542–74.
10. Wasilewski T, Kamysz W, Gębicki J. AI-assisted detection of biomarkers by sensors and biosensors for early diagnosis and monitoring. Biosensors. 2024;14(7):356.
11. Wang J, Lu X, He Y. Electrochemical detection of Tau proteins as biomarkers of Alzheimer's disease in blood. Biosensors. 2025;15(2):85.
12. Nan X, Wang X, Kang T, Zhang J, Dong L, Dong J, et al. Flexible wearable sensor devices for biomedical application: a review. Micromachines. 2022;13(9):1395.
13. Li L, Li Y, Pei J, Wu Y, Wang G, Zhang J, et al. Hotspots and trends of electrochemical biosensor technology: a bibliometric analysis (2003–2023). RSC Adv. 2023;13(44):30704–17.
14. Khan A, DeVoe E, Andreescu S. Carbon-based electrochemical biosensors as diagnostic platforms for decentralized healthcare. Sens Diagn. 2023;2(3):529–58.
15. Liu Y, Liu X, Wang X, Jiang H. AI-empowered electrochemical sensors for biomedical applications: advances and challenges. Biosensors. 2025;15(8):487.
16. Ates HC, Nguyen PQ, Gonzalez-Macia L, Morales-Narváez E, Güder F, Collins JJ, Dincer C. End-to-end design of wearable sensors. Nat Rev Mater. 2022;7(11):887–907.
17. Liu G, Yang Z. Insights in biosensors and biomolecular electronics 2024: developments, challenges, and perspectives. Front Bioeng Biotechnol. 2025;13:1668411.
18. Biswas SS, Mondal A, Kundu AK, Mandal P. Advancements in processing and manufacturing of nano-engineered materials: exploring nanotechnology applications in defence materials. In: Harmonising chemical and biological sciences for sustainable development; 2025.
19. Fu Y, Xia P, Chen C, Wang C, Zhang C, Zhang G, Feng S. Miniaturized 3D-printed ratiometric electrochemical immunosensing platform for ultrasensitive detection of depression biomarker Apo-A4. Talanta. 2025;284:127235.

20. Kumari SMNS, Suryabai XT. Sensing the future—frontiers in biosensors: classifications, principles, and advances. ACS Omega. 2024;9(50):48918–87.
21. Vo TS, Hoang T, Vo TTBC, Jeon B, Nguyen VH, Kim K. Bioanalytical sensors with smart health-monitoring systems: from materials to applications. Adv Healthc Mater. 2024;13(17):2303923.
22. Gideon O, Samuel HS, Okino IA. Biocompatible materials for next-generation biosensors. Discov Chem. 2024;1(1):34.
23. Baranwal A, Roy S, Kumar A. Nano-(bio)sensors for on-site monitoring: advancing diagnostics through technological intervention. Front Bioeng Biotechnol. 2024;12:1475130.
24. Dua A, Debnath A, Kumar K, Mazumder R, Mazumder A, Singh RK, et al. Advancements in glucose-monitoring biosensors: technological progress and innovation dynamics. Curr Pharm Biotechnol. 2025;26(11):1716–33.
25. Aihaiti A, Wang J, Zhang W, Shen M, Meng F, Li Z, et al. Innovative biosensor-based devices for heavy metal ion detection in food: recent advances and trends. Compr Rev Food Sci Food Saf. 2024;23(4):e13358.

Chapter 4
Review & Practice Problems

This chapter concludes the book with a focus on consolidation and self-assessment. Section 4.1 revisits the essential principles and applications of biosensors, summarizing major concepts such as sensor design, biorecognition mechanisms, signal transduction, and current technological developments. Section 4.2 complements this overview with multiple-choice questions aimed at reinforcing comprehension, testing key definitions, and strengthening analytical thinking. Together, these sections provide a structured review of biosensor fundamentals, supporting both exam preparation and deeper understanding of their biomedical relevance.

4.1 Summary of Key Concepts

Absolute error	Numerical difference between measured and true value, expressed in the same units as the measurand.
Accuracy	Closeness of measured value to the true analyte concentration.
Acoustic Biosensor	A Device that detects molecular interactions through variations in acoustic wave properties, such as frequency or velocity.
Adaptive biosensor	System capable of self-calibration, self-repair, or functional evolution through feedback mechanisms.
Affinity coupling	Immobilization through specific interactions such as biotin–streptavidin binding.
Affinity sensor	A Biosensor relying on reversible, non-catalytic binding interactions such as antibody–antigen or nucleic-acid hybridization.

© The Author(s), under exclusive license to Springer Nature Switzerland AG 2026

A. Badnjević, L. Spahić, *Biosensors*, Series in BioEngineering,
https://doi.org/10.1007/978-3-032-15757-7_4

AI-Driven Biosensing	Application of machine learning and deep learning algorithms for data interpretation and pattern recognition.
Amperometric biosensor	Device measuring current resulting from redox reactions at a fixed potential; current is proportional to analyte concentration.
Analog-to-digital converter (ADC)	Electronic device that converts continuous analog signals into discrete digital values.
Analyte	Substance being detected or quantified by a biosensor.
Analytical validation	Process confirming biosensor accuracy, precision, linearity, and stability under practical conditions.
Anomaly Detection	AI-based identification of irregular or unexpected biosensor signal patterns.
Antigen–Antibody Complex	Specific binding pair forming the basis of immunosensor recognition.
Aptamer	Short DNA or RNA oligonucleotide binding targets with high specificity and affinity.
Artificial Pancreas	Closed-loop system integrating glucose sensors with insulin pumps for automated diabetes control.
Autonomous Decision Support	Intelligent biosensor capability to predict physiological changes and recommend interventions.
Baseline Correction	Data-processing method that removes background signal before analysis.
Biocatalytic sensor	Biosensor using enzymatic or metabolic reactions to convert analytes into measurable electrochemical signals.
Biocompatibility	Ability of a biosensor to function in contact with biological tissue without eliciting adverse reactions.
Biodegradable biosensor	Environmentally friendly sensor made from materials that decompose naturally after use.
Bioelectrochemical transduction	Conversion of biochemical reaction energy into measurable electrical output via electron or ion transfer.
BioFET (Biological Field-Effect Transistor)	Semiconductor-based biosensor detecting charge variations caused by biological interactions.
Biofouling	Unwanted accumulation of biological material on sensor surfaces, leading to signal drift or degradation.

Biofouling resistance	Surface property preventing nonspecific adsorption of biomolecules that degrade sensor performance.
Bioimaging Nanomaterial	Nanostructure emitting optical signals for non-invasive imaging of biological tissues.
Biomedical Biosensor	Analytical device detecting physiological or biochemical changes within the human body for diagnostic or monitoring purposes.
Biomimetic sensor	Synthetic sensor that mimics biological recognition, often through molecularly imprinted polymers (MIPs).
Bioreceptor	Biological molecule (enzyme, antibody, nucleic acid, cell, or receptor) that recognizes and binds the target analyte.
Biorecognition element (Bio-receptor)	The biological component (enzyme, antibody, nucleic acid, cell, or tissue) responsible for specific analyte recognition.
Bioresorbable Sensor	Implantable device designed to dissolve harmlessly after use within biological tissues.
Biosensor	Analytical device that combines a biological recognition element with a transducer to detect and quantify chemical or biological analytes.
Black phosphorus (BP)	2D semiconductor with tunable bandgap offering superior sensitivity in nanoscale biosensing.
Calibration Algorithm	Software function adjusting readings to maintain accuracy under variable conditions.
Calibration certificate	Official document reporting the calibration result and associated uncertainty for an instrument or reference material.
Calibration curve	Graphical relationship between known analyte concentrations and sensor response used to determine unknown samples.
Calibration function	Mathematical relationship linking sensor input and output under standard conditions.
Calibration hierarchy	Sequence of calibration steps linking laboratory instruments to national or international measurement standards.
Calibration slope and intercept	Parameters defining the linear relationship between biosensor signal and analyte concentration, each contributing to total uncertainty.

Capacitance (C_{ox})	Charge storage per unit voltage across the dielectric; inversely affects voltage shift sensitivity.
CE marking	Certification indicating conformity with EU health, safety, and environmental standards for marketed devices.
Cell-based biosensor	Sensor employing living cells or tissues to detect physiological or toxic responses.
Cell-Based FET	Device using live cells to monitor physiological responses via electrical modulation.
Central limit theorem	Statistical principle stating that the sum of many random variables tends toward a normal distribution.
Certified reference material (CRM)	Reference material accompanied by a certificate establishing its value and uncertainty traceable to SI units.
Channel Material	Semiconductor medium (e.g., silicon, graphene, MoS_2) where charge conduction occurs.
Charge-Transfer Resistance (Rct)	Resistance to electron transfer between electrode and analyte; indicator of binding efficiency.
Chi-square ($\chi2$) distribution	Statistical model describing sums of squared standardized deviations, used to assess variance.
Cholesterol biosensor	Amperometric device using cholesterol oxidase to oxidize cholesterol and detect resulting hydrogen peroxide.
Chronoamperometry (CA)	Technique where a step potential is applied and current is recorded over time to study reaction rates.
Clark enzyme electrode	The first modern biosensor (1962) developed by Leland Clark, using glucose oxidase and a platinum oxygen electrode for glucose detection.
Colorimetric Detection	Measurement based on color change resulting from analyte interaction or nanoparticle aggregation.
Combined standard uncertainty	Overall uncertainty of a result obtained by combining the standard uncertainties of all input quantities according to the propagation law.

Comparability	Capability of relating results from different instruments or laboratories through traceable and uncertainty-qualified measurements.
Compensatory technique	Method that neutralizes systematic bias during measurement through reversal or substitution.
Conductometric biosensor	Sensor detecting analyte-induced variations in electrical conductivity of a medium.
Confidence interval	Range around a measured value within which the true value is expected to lie with a given probability.
Continuous Glucose Monitoring (CGM)	System that measures glucose levels in interstitial fluid at regular intervals for diabetes management.
Conventional true value	Experimentally established approximation used as a substitute for the inaccessible true value.
Correction procedure	Post-measurement adjustment applied to compensate for identified systematic errors.
Correlated quantities	Input parameters whose variations are statistically dependent, requiring covariance consideration in uncertainty combination.
Correlation coefficient	Statistical measure describing the strength of dependence between two variables in calibration data.
Counter (or auxiliary) electrode	Electrode that completes the circuit, balancing current flow within the electrochemical cell.
Covalent bonding	Chemical attachment of biomolecules using cross-linkers for stable immobilization.
Covariance term	Statistical term representing correlation between two input quantities; included when inputs are not independent.
Coverage factor (k)	Numerical multiplier used to scale the standard uncertainty to a desired confidence level (e.g., $k = 2 \approx 95\%$).
Coverage probability (p)	Probability that the true value lies within the range $y \pm U$ of the measurement result.
C-Reactive Protein (CRP) Biosensor	Diagnostic sensor detecting CRP as an early indicator of infection or inflammation.
CRISPR-Cas Biosensor	Genetic detection tool employing CRISPR-associated enzymes for specific nucleic acid recognition and cleavage.

Cybersecurity in biosensing	Implementation of encryption and secure data protocols to protect patient or analytical information in connected biosensors.
Cyclic voltammetry (CV)	Electrochemical method involving cyclic potential sweeps to examine redox behavior and reaction kinetics.
Damping ratio (ξ)	Parameter describing how oscillations decay; determines whether the system is underdamped, critically damped, or overdamped.
Data Privacy in Wearables	Protection of sensitive biometric data transmitted by connected biosensing devices.
Decision-oriented reporting	Expression of uncertainty in clear, user-relevant terms (e.g., probability that true analyte concentration lies within a given range).
Degrees of freedom (v)	Number of independent data points used to estimate variability (typically $n - 1$ for n observations).
Diagnostic Biosensor	Device used to identify diseases by detecting specific biomarkers such as enzymes, antibodies, or nucleic acids.
Dielectric Layer	Insulating layer separating the gate from the channel, determining capacitance and sensitivity.
Digital-to-analog converter (DAC)	Circuit that converts digital data back into analog form for output or control.
Direct monitoring	Biosensing mode in which the analyte itself is measured electrochemically.
Disposable biosensor	Single-use biosensor designed for sterile, rapid measurements where reusability is impractical.
DNA (or nucleic acid) biosensor	Device detecting complementary sequence hybridization events via electrical or optical signal changes.
DNA-FET (GenFET)	FET biosensor employing DNA probes for hybridization-based nucleic acid detection.
Documentation of uncertainty	Detailed record including measurement model, input list, uncertainty evaluations, and final uncertainty statement for audit or publication.
Drift	Gradual change in baseline sensor output over time without change in input.
Dynamic characteristics	Parameters defining sensor behavior when subjected to time-varying inputs.

Dynamic error	Deviation caused by finite response time when input changes rapidly.
Dynamic range	Range of analyte concentrations over which the sensor response remains linear.
Eco-Design of Biosensors	Development of recyclable or biodegradable biosensors minimizing environmental impact.
Edge AI Processing	On-device computation of biosensor data without relying on cloud connectivity.
Effective degrees of freedom ($v_e$ff)	Weighted estimate of total statistical confidence across multiple uncertainty components, calculated by the Welch–Satterthwaite equation.
Electrochemical biosensor	Analytical device that converts a biological recognition event into an electrical signal through redox or ion-transfer processes at an electrode interface.
Electrochemical impedance spectroscopy (EIS)	Technique analyzing system impedance over varying frequencies to study electrode kinetics and interface properties.
Electrochemical Patch	Flexible biosensor employing electrochemical detection principles for noninvasive monitoring.
Electrochemical transduction	Signal generation based on current, voltage, or impedance changes.
Electron transfer kinetics	Rate and mechanism by which electrons move between analyte, mediator, and electrode.
Energy Harvesting	Technique of powering biosensors using environmental or physiological energy sources such as heat or motion.
Entrapment	Encapsulation of bioreceptors within polymeric or sol–gel matrices.
Environmental traceability	Calibration and documentation of environmental parameters (temperature, pH, humidity) influencing biosensor response.
Enzyme-based biosensor	Sensor utilizing enzymatic catalysis to convert analytes into measurable products.
Equivalent Circuit Model	Electrical representation of electrochemical interfaces using resistors, capacitors, and diffusion elements.
Error	Difference between the measured value and the true or reference value.

Error vs. uncertainty	Error is the deviation from the true value; uncertainty expresses the range in which the true value likely lies.
Ethical Biosensing	Framework ensuring privacy, consent, and responsible data handling in biosensor use.
Expanded uncertainty (U)	Standard uncertainty multiplied by a coverage factor k to provide an interval containing a specified proportion of possible true values.
Experimental mean ($\bar{x}$)	Arithmetic average of repeated measurements representing the best estimate of a quantity.
Experimental variance (s2)	Measure of dispersion among repeated readings, calculated from deviations from the mean.
Faradaic Process	Electrochemical reaction involving charge transfer across the electrode interface.
F-distribution (Fisher distribution)	Describes ratio of two variances; used to compare dispersion between datasets.
Feature Extraction	Computational process identifying key signal parameters for quantitative analysis.
Fiducial error	Ratio of absolute error to the instrument's full-scale value, used to express specification limits.
Field-effect transduction	Signal produced by charge variations at a semiconductor interface.
Field-Effect Transistor (FET)	Semiconductor device controlling current via an electric field applied to a gate electrode.
First-order system	Sensor model with exponential response characterized by a single time constant (τ).
Fluorescence biosensor	Sensor using light emission from fluorophores to detect analyte presence or binding events.
Fluorescence resonance energy transfer (FRET)	Distance-dependent energy transfer between donor and acceptor fluorophores used for quantitative sensing.
Foreign Body Response	Immune reaction leading to encapsulation or inflammation around implanted sensors.
Frequency analysis	Evaluation of signal components based on their frequencies to identify patterns or interference.
Frequency Shift (Δf)	Change in oscillation frequency proportional to mass or viscosity change on a QCM/SAW surface.

Functionalization	Chemical modification of a nanomaterial surface to enable biomolecule immobilization and biocompatibility.
Galvanostat	Device that maintains a constant current in an electrochemical cell while monitoring the corresponding potential changes.
Generalized normal distribution	Modified Gaussian distribution including a shape parameter to accommodate skewed or peaked data.
Genosensor (DNA/RNA Biosensor)	Biosensor that identifies specific nucleotide sequences to detect genetic mutations or pathogens.
Giant magnetoresistance (GMR) biosensor	Magnetic sensor based on resistance changes in multilayer ferromagnetic structures upon analyte binding.
Good Clinical Practice (GCP)	Regulatory standard ensuring ethical and scientific quality in clinical trials.
Graphene and 2D materials	High-mobility, large-surface-area materials improving FET-biosensor performance and miniaturization.
Gross error	Large, identifiable mistake from misreading, equipment malfunction, or procedural faults.
Hexagonal boron nitride (h-BN)	Two-dimensional dielectric material enhancing stability and insulation in FET-based biosensors.
Hybrid biosensor	System combining multiple transduction modes (e.g., electrochemical + optical) for enhanced performance or multiplex detection.
Hydroxyapatite Nanoparticle	Bioceramic additive used to enhance mechanical strength in bone tissue scaffolds.
Hysteresis	Difference in sensor output for the same input depending on input direction (increasing or decreasing).
IEC 60601 series	International standards specifying electrical safety and electromagnetic compatibility of medical equipment.
Immobilization	Method of fixing biological recognition elements onto a sensor surface using adsorption, covalent bonding, or encapsulation.
Immunosensor	Device that uses antigen–antibody specificity for target detection.

Impedance	Complex resistance combining resistive and reactive components of an electrochemical system under AC excitation.
Impedimetric biosensor	Sensor evaluating changes in impedance at an electrode interface, often used for label-free detection.
Implantable biosensor	Miniaturized, biocompatible sensor designed for in-body monitoring of biochemical parameters.
Indirect monitoring	Measurement of a compound that affects the biological recognition element (e.g., inhibitor or activator).
Inductive Coupling	Wireless power or data transmission technique using electromagnetic induction.
Influence quantity	Factor other than the measurand that affects the measurement outcome (e.g., temperature, pH, electrode condition).
Instrumental error	Deviation caused by imperfections or limitations of measuring devices.
Intelligent bioprocessing	Integration of biosensors with machine learning for real-time process optimization in biotechnology.
Interaction error	Error arising when the measuring device influences the object being measured.
Interdigital Transducer (IDT)	Electrode structure that converts electrical signals into acoustic waves and vice versa in SAW sensors.
Interferometric Biosensor	Device measuring phase or intensity shifts from interference of light reflected by sensing and reference surfaces.
Intrinsic error	Systematic deviation inherent to instrument design or normal operation.
Ion-selective electrode (ISE)	Electrochemical sensor that selectively responds to a particular ion through a selective membrane.
Ion-Sensitive FET (ISFET)	FET variant with ion-sensitive membrane detecting ion concentration changes.
IoT biosensor	Sensor connected to Internet-of-Things networks for continuous data transmission and remote monitoring.
ISO 13485	International standard for quality management in medical device manufacturing.
ISO 14971	Standard governing risk management for medical-device design and manufacturing.

ISO 15197	Standard specifying performance requirements for blood glucose monitoring systems.
ISO GUM (Guide to the Expression of Uncertainty in Measurement)	International standard providing principles and procedures for evaluating and expressing measurement uncertainty.
ISO/IEC 17025	Standard outlining competence requirements for testing and calibration laboratories.
IUPAC biosensor criteria	Standardized performance definitions including calibration range, sensitivity, linearity, detection limit, selectivity, stability, and response time.
IVDR (In Vitro Diagnostic Regulation)	EU regulation governing diagnostic device approval and post-market surveillance.
IVDR 2017/746	EU regulation establishing conformity assessment and performance evaluation requirements for in-vitro diagnostic devices.
Knowledge Distillation	Process of compressing large AI models into smaller, efficient forms suitable for portable biosensors.
Label-Free Detection	Analytical method measuring direct interactions without fluorescent or radioactive markers.
Lab-on-a-Chip	Miniaturized system integrating multiple laboratory functions on a single microdevice.
Lactate biosensor	Amperometric sensor employing lactate oxidase or dehydrogenase to quantify lactate levels as indicators of metabolic activity.
Law of propagation of uncertainty	Mathematical rule using partial derivatives to calculate how input-quantity uncertainties affect the output uncertainty.
Limit of Detection (LOD)	Lowest analyte concentration distinguishable from background noise.
Linear time-invariant (LTI) system	System with proportional (linear) and time-independent behavior; used for modeling sensor dynamics.
Linearity	Degree to which the sensor's response is directly proportional to analyte concentration (measured via R^2).
Liquid-Gated FET	FET configuration where gate voltage is applied through an electrolyte using a reference electrode.

Magnetic biosensor	Device that detects analyte-induced magnetic-field variations using magnetic nanoparticles or thin-film structures.
Magnetic particle spectroscopy (MPS)	Technique analyzing the magnetic response of particle-bound analytes for label-free detection.
Mass Loading Effect	Frequency decrease caused by the addition of analyte mass on the piezoelectric surface.
Mass transport	Movement of analyte to the electrode surface via diffusion or convection influencing current response.
Material Sustainability	Design approach ensuring biosensor components are renewable, recyclable, or degradable.
Matrix effect	Interference caused by complex sample components that affect sensor accuracy.
Mean (μ)	Average of measured values representing the central tendency of data.
Measurand	Specific physical or chemical quantity intended to be measured, clearly defined to avoid ambiguity (e.g., glucose concentration in whole blood at 37 °C).
Measurement certainty	Level of confidence that a measurement result meets its intended precision and reliability requirements.
Measurement confidence level	Statistical probability (commonly 95%) that the true value lies within the reported uncertainty interval.
Measurement model	Mathematical relationship linking the measurand to input quantities that influence it.
Measurement range (span)	Range between the smallest and largest measurable values that maintain accuracy.
Measurement uncertainty	Quantitative estimate describing the range within which the true value is expected to lie.
Methodological error	Error resulting from inadequacies in measurement technique or model assumptions.
Metrological characteristics	Quantitative parameters defining an instrument's precision, accuracy, and stability.
Microfluidic biosensor	Miniaturized device that manipulates microliter-scale fluids through microchannels for integrated sample processing and sensing.
Microfluidics	Technology for manipulating fluids at the microscale, enabling lab-on-a-chip biosensors.

Microscale Biosensor	Miniaturized sensor operating with small sample volumes and high detection efficiency.
Miniaturization	Reduction of biosensor size through micro-fabrication and nanotechnology for portable or wearable applications.
Minimum detectable signal (MDS)	Lowest measurable signal distinguishable from background noise; also called detection threshold.
Molecularly imprinted polymer (MIP)	Artificial polymer with recognition sites complementary to a target molecule's shape and functionality.
Monoclonal Antibody	Single-specificity antibody used for precise antigen recognition.
Multiplex Immunosensor	Device capable of detecting multiple bio-markers in parallel.
Multiplexed Biosensing	Simultaneous detection of multiple analytes within a single device or platform.
Nanocomposite Scaffold	Hybrid polymeric material reinforced with nanoparticles for tissue engineering applications.
Nanomaterial	Material with nanoscale features used to enhance surface area, conductivity, or optical signal strength.
Nanostructured electrode	Electrode modified with nanomaterials (e.g., CNTs, graphene) to increase surface area and electron-transfer efficiency.
Nanotoxicity	Potential harmful biological effects of nanoparticles introduced into the body.
Natural frequency (ω)	Frequency at which an undamped system oscillates after a disturbance.
Nernst equation	Relationship describing electrode potential as a function of temperature and reactant/product concentrations.
Next-generation biosensor	Integrated, miniaturized, multifunctional device combining microelectronics, AI-assisted data processing, and smart connectivity.
Noise	Unwanted fluctuation in sensor output unrelated to the measured signal.
Normal (Gaussian) distribution	Symmetrical probability distribution describing random errors centered around the mean.

Normalization
(of metrological characteristics)   Standardization of instrument parameters to ensure consistent accuracy and performance.

Nyquist Plot   Graph displaying real vs. imaginary impedance components for EIS data interpretation.

Operational stability   Retention of sensor performance over repeated use or storage.

Optical Immunosensor   Sensor detecting optical property changes such as fluorescence or refractive index.

Optical transduction   Measurement through light absorption, fluorescence, or surface plasmon resonance.

Overshoot   Extent to which a transient response exceeds its final steady value.

Parallel Computing (GPU/TPU)   Hardware acceleration method enabling rapid AI-driven data analysis in biosensor systems.

Photoelectrochemical biosensor   Hybrid system coupling light-activated semiconductors with biological recognition elements to generate photocurrents.

Photonic Crystal Biosensor   Sensor using periodic dielectric structures to detect refractive-index changes upon analyte binding.

Photoplethysmography (PPG)   Optical technique measuring changes in blood volume to determine heart rate and oxygen saturation.

Physical adsorption   Weak binding of bioreceptors through van der Waals or hydrophobic interactions.

Piezoelectric (acoustic) transduction   Detection of mass or frequency changes on a crystal surface.

Point-of-care (POC) testing   Diagnostic testing conducted near the patient or sample source for rapid results.

Polarization   Orientation or phase alteration of light upon interaction with analyte or surface.

Polyclonal Antibody   Mixture of antibodies recognizing multiple epitopes on a target antigen.

Post-Market Clinical Follow-Up
(PMCF)   Continued clinical evaluation after device approval to confirm long-term safety.

Post-Market Surveillance (PMS)   Continuous monitoring of device performance and safety after commercialization.

Potentiometric biosensor   Device that measures potential differences caused by ionic activity changes near an ion-

	selective electrode under negligible current flow.
Potentiostat	Instrument that maintains a controlled potential between working and reference electrodes and measures the resulting current.
Precision	Degree of repeatability among multiple measurements under unchanged conditions.
Premarket Approval (PMA)	FDA pathway requiring clinical data for high-risk medical device authorization.
Preventive Biosensing	Use of biosensors for early detection of disease risks before symptom onset.
Preventive error control	Pre-measurement measures like thermal stabilization or shielding to minimize systematic error sources.
Principal Component Analysis (PCA)	Statistical technique reducing dimensionality to visualize biosensor data trends.
Quality assurance in biosensing	Application of standardized uncertainty evaluation, traceability, and reporting practices to ensure reliability and regulatory compliance.
Quantum Dot Sensor	Optical biosensor using nanoscale semiconductors for fluorescent signal generation.
Quartz Crystal Microbalance (QCM)	Piezoelectric sensor measuring minute mass changes via shifts in resonant frequency.
Raman Spectroscopy	Optical method detecting inelastic light scattering that reveals molecular vibrational information.
Randles Circuit	Equivalent circuit model including solution resistance, double-layer capacitance, charge-transfer resistance, and diffusion impedance.
Random error	Unpredictable deviation in measurements due to uncontrollable fluctuations.
Random variable	Quantity whose possible values result from random phenomena, described by a probability distribution.
Rare-Earth Doped Nanomaterial	Luminescent nanomaterial used for bioimaging and fluorescence-based sensing.
Reaction quotient (Q)	Ratio of product to reactant concentrations used in the Nernst equation.
Reaction–Transport Kinetics	Rate at which analytes diffuse to and react at the sensor surface, affecting sensitivity.
Recovery time	Duration for sensor output to return to baseline after removal of stimulus.

Rectangular (uniform) distribution	Probability model assuming all values within a range are equally likely; standard uncertainty = $a/\sqrt{3}$.
Redox reaction	Chemical process involving simultaneous oxidation and reduction; fundamental to electrochemical detection.
Reference electrode	Electrode providing a stable, well-defined potential against which the working-electrode potential is measured.
Reinforcement Learning	AI training approach optimizing biosensor signal interpretation through iterative feedback.
Relative error	Ratio of absolute error to the true value, typically expressed as a percentage.
Relative standard uncertainty	Standard uncertainty expressed as a fraction of the measured value; used for proportional uncertainty comparisons.
Remote Monitoring	Continuous tracking of health parameters via wireless data transmission to healthcare systems.
Repeatability	Ability of a sensor to produce the same reading under identical, repeated conditions.
Reproducibility	Ability to produce consistent results under identical conditions.
Residual systematic error	Remaining bias after correction; estimated theoretically when direct measurement is impossible.
Resolution (discrimination)	Smallest detectable input change that produces a measurable change in output.
Response Time	Duration between analyte introduction and measurable signal generation.
Rise time	Interval needed for output to move from 10% to 90% of its final value in a dynamic response.
Root-sum-square (RSS) method	Statistical approach for combining independent uncertainty components.
Rounding protocol	Practice of rounding values only after uncertainty combination to prevent compounding rounding errors.
Sauerbrey Equation	Relationship between frequency shift and mass change in a QCM sensor surface ($\Delta f = -C\Delta m$).
Second-order system	Model describing sensors that may exhibit oscillatory or damped responses.

Selectivity	Ability of a biosensor to distinguish the target analyte from interfering substances.
Self-healing materials	Surface coatings capable of restoring structural or functional integrity after minor damage to prolong sensor lifespan.
Self-powered biosensor	Device that generates its own operational energy from biochemical reactions or body heat.
Sensitivity	Minimum detectable concentration of an analyte.
Sensitivity coefficient	Quantitative measure of how a change in an influencing factor affects measurement output.
Settling time	Time required for output to remain within a specified error band around its final value.
SI unit traceability	Assurance that measurements are expressed in units of the International System (e.g., mol L−1, V, A).
Signal amplifier and processor	Electronic components that enhance and interpret weak electrochemical signals into readable outputs.
Signal Drift	Gradual change in sensor output due to aging, fouling, or environmental variations.
Signal processing	Operations applied to raw sensor output to enhance accuracy, reduce noise, and extract meaningful data.
Signal stability	Consistency of output over repeated or long-term operation, critical for continuous monitoring applications.
Signal Transduction	Conversion of biological interactions into electrical signals measurable by the FET circuit.
Signal-to-noise ratio (S/N)	Ratio of signal mean to noise standard deviation; higher values indicate cleaner signals.
Single-Use (Disposable) Biosensor	Sensor intended for one-time measurement to prevent contamination or cross-reactivity.
Smart biosensor	Advanced biosensor integrating AI or microcontrollers for real-time data processing and autonomous decision-making.
Software (Firmware)	Control and data-processing program managing measurement, calibration, and visualization in biosensor systems.
Solution Resistance (Rs)	Ohmic resistance of electrolyte solution between electrodes.

Specificity	Ability to distinguish the target analyte from similar substances.
Stability	Ability of a sensor to maintain consistent performance over time with minimal drift.
Standard deviation (σ)	Square root of variance; measure of data dispersion and uncertainty.
Standard uncertainty (u)	Uncertainty expressed as a standard deviation; the most basic quantitative expression of uncertainty.
Standard uncertainty of the mean ($u(\bar{x})$)	Uncertainty of the average value, calculated as $s/\sqrt{n}$.
Static characteristics	Sensor parameters describing steady-state behavior under unchanging conditions.
Static sensitivity (K)	Constant ratio between output and input in a zero-order system.
Student's t-distribution	Probability model for small-sample means when population variance is unknown.
Subjective error	Error introduced by human observation or interpretation.
Supplemental error	Error caused by environmental deviations such as temperature or humidity changes.
Support Vector Machine (SVM)	Machine learning model used for classification of biosensor responses.
Surface Acoustic Wave (SAW) Sensor	Device using acoustic waves propagating along a substrate surface to detect mass or viscoelastic changes.
Surface Functionalization	Modification of electrode or optical substrate to enable bioreceptor attachment and reduce nonspecific binding.
Surface Plasmon Resonance (SPR)	Optical technique measuring refractive index changes at a metal surface during binding events.
Surface-to-Volume Ratio	Geometric property influencing the sensitivity and reactivity of nanoscale and microscale sensors.
Sustainability in biosensing	Design approach emphasizing recyclable materials, energy efficiency, and minimal environmental impact.
Sweat Biosensor	Wearable device analyzing biochemical components such as glucose, lactate, or cortisol in sweat.

Systematic error	Predictable deviation that consistently biases measurement results; often correctable by calibration.
Telemedicine Integration	Incorporation of biosensor data into digital healthcare networks for remote clinical decision-making.
Therapeutic Drug Monitoring (TDM)	Measurement of drug concentrations in biological fluids to optimize dosage and minimize toxicity.
Thermal transduction	Detection of heat generated or absorbed during biochemical reactions.
Time constant (τ)	Time needed for a first-order system's output to reach about 63% of its final value after a step input.
Traceability	Property of a measurement result whereby it can be related to reference standards through an unbroken chain of comparisons, each with stated uncertainty.
Transducer	Physical component that converts a biological or chemical event into a measurable electrical, optical, or mechanical signal.
Transition metal dichalcogenides (TMDCs)	Layered semiconductors (e.g., MoS_2) used in high-sensitivity field-effect transducers.
Triangular distribution	Probability model assuming central values are more likely than extreme ones; standard uncertainty = $a/\sqrt{6}$.
Tumor Biomarker	Biological molecule indicating the presence or progression of cancer (e.g., PSA, CEA, HER2).
Type A uncertainty evaluation	Statistical determination of uncertainty based on repeated measurements and analysis of variance.
Type B uncertainty evaluation	Estimation of uncertainty using non-statistical information such as calibration data, literature values, or expert judgment.
Uncertainty budget	Structured tabulation of all sources of uncertainty, their values, evaluation methods, and mathematical combination leading to $u_{(c)}$ and U.
Urease biosensor	Device employing urease to hydrolyze urea into ammonia and bicarbonate, enabling potentiometric detection.
Variance ($\sigma2$)	Average of squared deviations from the mean, indicating data spread.

Viscoelastic Property — Combined viscous and elastic behavior of materials affecting acoustic wave propagation.

Voltammetric biosensor — Device measuring current as the potential is swept over time to characterize oxidation-reduction behavior.

Warburg Impedance — Frequency-dependent impedance element representing diffusion-controlled processes.

Wearable Biosensor — Flexible device designed for continuous, noninvasive monitoring of physiological biomarkers.

Welch–Satterthwaite equation — Formula used to compute v_{eff} for combined uncertainty components with differing variances and sample sizes.

Wireless SAW Sensor — Passive, battery-free sensor using reflected acoustic signals for remote monitoring.

Working electrode — Primary electrode where the biochemical reaction occurs and the signal is generated.

Zero-order system — Ideal sensor with instantaneous response and no delay between input and output.

4.2   Practice Problems and Exercises

4.2.1   *Introduction to Biosensors*

1. According to IUPAC, a biosensor must include which two essential components?

    a) Bioreceptor and indicator dye
    b) Biological recognition element and transducer
    c) Catalyst and reference electrode
    d) Reagent and cuvette

2. The function of the biological recognition element is to:

    a) Amplify electrical signals
    b) Detect physical changes in electrodes
    c) Provide specific binding or catalytic activity toward the analyte
    d) Store calibration data

3. The first modern biosensor was developed by Leland C. Clark Jr. to detect:

    a) Oxygen in blood
    b) Glucose concentration
    c) Urea in urine
    d) Lactate in muscle tissue

4. In Clark's original enzyme electrode, oxygen concentration decreased because:

    a) The enzyme consumed glucose
    b) Glucose oxidase used oxygen as an electron acceptor
    c) Oxygen reacted with platinum
    d) Hydrogen peroxide was reduced to oxygen

5. Which immobilization method uses van der Waals or hydrophobic forces?

    a) Covalent bonding
    b) Entrapment
    c) Physical adsorption
    d) Affinity coupling

6. The sensitivity of a biosensor is mathematically expressed as:

    a) $S = 3\sigma/C$
    b) $S = \Delta Y/\Delta C$
    c) $S = \Delta C/\Delta Y$
    d) $S = \sigma \times Y$

7. A sensor that measures the change in refractive index upon binding events operates on which transduction principle?

    a) Electrochemical
    b) Piezoelectric
    c) Optical
    d) Thermal

8. The limit of detection (LOD) is calculated using the formula:

    a) $LOD = S/\sigma$
    b) $LOD = 3\sigma/S$
    c) $LOD = \sigma/3S$
    d) $LOD = 1/(3\sigma S)$

9. Which ISO standard specifies requirements for glucose monitoring systems?

    a) ISO 13485
    b) ISO 15197
    c) ISO/IEC 17025
    d) ISO 9001

10. Molecularly imprinted polymers (MIPs) are used because they:

    a) Are living cells that sense pH changes
    b) Contain synthetic recognition sites complementary to analytes
    c) Are enzymes with higher catalytic turnover
    d) Provide electrochemical amplification

11. A glucose biosensor exhibits a linear range from 0.1 mM to 10 mM. What happens when glucose concentration exceeds 10 mM?

a) Sensitivity increases
b) Enzyme becomes saturated and linearity is lost
c) Signal becomes independent of oxygen concentration
d) Calibration curve remains unchanged

12. A cell-based biosensor detects heavy metals through the inhibited respiration of microorganisms. What type of transduction is most suitable?

a) Thermal
b) Electrochemical (amperometric)
c) Optical fluorescence
d) Piezoelectric resonance

13. A biosensor shows the following data for glucose concentration and signal output:

Glucose (mM)	Signal (μA)
0.5	0.8
1.0	1.6
1.5	2.4
2.0	3.2

Calculate the sensor sensitivity ($S = \Delta Y / \Delta C$).

14. If the standard deviation of the blank (σ) is 0.02 μA and the sensitivity (S) is 1.6 μA mM^{-1}, find the LOD ($LOD = 3\sigma/S$).

15. Explain why nanomaterials such as gold nanoparticles or graphene can enhance biosensor sensitivity.

4.2.2 Foundations of Biosensors

1. Biomedical biosensors are primarily used to:

a) Detect mechanical vibrations
b) Measure biological or chemical changes in living systems
c) Analyze structural materials in engineering
d) Monitor light intensity in optical fibers

2. The earliest biomedical biosensor successfully commercialized was designed for:

a) Detecting blood oxygen
b) Monitoring blood glucose levels
c) Measuring lactic acid in muscles
d) Estimating cholesterol in plasma

3. The biological recognition element in a glucose biosensor is typically:

   a) Urease
   b) Lactate oxidase
   c) Glucose oxidase
   d) Peroxidase

4. Continuous glucose monitoring systems (CGMs) operate by:

   a) Detecting pH variations in the bloodstream
   b) Measuring the rate of glucose oxidation in interstitial fluid
   c) Using antibodies to bind to insulin
   d) Counting red blood cells electrochemically

5. Electrochemical biosensors used in medical diagnostics are favored because they:

   a) Have very low power consumption and easy miniaturization
   b) Require bulky optical equipment
   c) Operate only under vacuum
   d) Depend solely on mechanical deformation

6. Which of the following best describes an immunosensor?

   a) A biosensor based on enzyme catalysis
   b) A biosensor based on antigen–antibody interaction
   c) A biosensor using cell metabolism
   d) A biosensor employing DNA hybridization

7. Optical biosensors are particularly valuable in biomedicine because they:

   a) Can detect analytes without electrical contact
   b) Always require fluorescent labeling
   c) Are immune to temperature variation
   d) Cannot be miniaturized

8. Which of the following is *not* a biomedical application of biosensors?

   a) Monitoring patient glucose
   b) Detection of disease biomarkers
   c) Food freshness detection in packaging
   d) Continuous blood pressure measurement

9. The main advantage of wearable biosensors is:

   a) Single-use capability only
   b) Continuous, non-invasive monitoring
   c) Dependence on laboratory calibration every hour
   d) High cost and low portability

10. Biosensors used for detecting infectious diseases often rely on:

    a) Spectrophotometric analysis of culture media
    b) Electrochemical immunoassays
    c) Radiolabeled tracers
    d) Mass spectrometric ionization

11. A biosensor for cardiac biomarker detection would most likely use:

    a) Enzyme–substrate interaction
    b) Antibody–antigen binding
    c) DNA hybridization
    d) Thermal gradient sensing

12. Point-of-care biosensors are designed to:

    a) Replace surgical diagnostic tools
    b) Enable testing at or near the site of patient care
    c) Eliminate the need for calibration
    d) Require high-voltage operation

13. In a lactate biosensor, which reaction is primarily measured?

    a) Lactate $\rightarrow$ Pyruvate + H_2O_2
    b) Pyruvate $\rightarrow$ Lactate + ATP
    c) Lactate + O_2 $\rightarrow$ CO_2 + H_2O
    d) Lactate $\rightarrow$ Glucose + NADH

14. The signal from an electrochemical glucose biosensor is typically proportional to:

    a) Oxygen evolution
    b) Hydrogen ion consumption
    c) Hydrogen peroxide formation
    d) Temperature gradient

15. In continuous glucose monitors, enzyme degradation over time affects:

    a) Sensitivity and stability
    b) Linearity only
    c) Response time only
    d) Signal polarity

16. In monitoring sepsis biomarkers, biosensors should primarily ensure:

    a) Rapid response and high sensitivity at low concentrations
    b) Slow response to minimize noise
    c) High operating temperature
    d) Constant sample stirring

17. A DNA biosensor that detects a specific viral genome works based on:

    a) Complementary base pairing
    b) Enzyme catalysis
    c) Protein folding
    d) Cell respiration

18. A biosensor for detecting cortisol in sweat should focus primarily on optimizing:

    a) Biocompatibility and signal stability
    b) Colorimetric reaction rate
    c) Electrical resistance of electrodes
    d) Gas permeability of membranes

19. In a typical enzyme-based biosensor, enzyme immobilization improves:

    a) Specificity, reusability, and stability
    b) Color visualization
    c) Sample dilution
    d) Thermal interference

20. The performance of biomedical biosensors can degrade in real samples due to:

    a) Matrix effects and non-specific adsorption
    b) Constant calibration
    c) Reduced diffusion in standard buffers
    d) Controlled laboratory conditions

4.2.3   Uncertainty in Sensor Measurements

1. Measurement precision refers to:

    a) Agreement between measured and true values
    b) Reproducibility of repeated measurements
    c) Ability to measure very small quantities
    d) Correction of systematic deviations

2. The term measurement certainty means:

    a) The result is exact and error-free
    b) The result is sufficiently precise for its intended purpose
    c) The result has zero deviation
    d) The result is verified by two independent laboratories

3. The true value of a physical quantity:

    a) Can be determined exactly with ideal instruments
    b) Is estimated experimentally but never known precisely

   c) Equals the arithmetic mean of many readings
   d) Is the nominal value from the instrument's scale

4. The measurement error ΔX is defined as:

   a) $\Delta X = X - X_{tr}$
   b) $\Delta X = X_{tr} - X$
   c) $\Delta X = X/X_{tr}$
   d) $\Delta X = (X + X_{tr})/2$

5. A measurement result reported with uncertainty should include:

   a) Only the mean value
   b) The probable range and confidence level
   c) The largest single reading
   d) No indication of precision

6. Absolute error is expressed in:

   a) Percent of true value
   b) The same units as the measured quantity
   c) Arbitrary units
   d) Relative terms only

7. Relative error represents:

   a) The ratio of absolute error to true or measured value
   b) The square of the absolute error
   c) The calibration offset
   d) The average deviation per second

8. Which of the following is not a source-based classification of error?

   a) Instrumental error
   b) Methodological error
   c) Subjective error
   d) Statistical error

9. Subjective errors arise mainly from:

   a) Imperfect mathematical models
   b) Operator perception and reaction limits
   c) Temperature fluctuations
   d) Calibration drift

10. Systematic errors differ from random errors because they:

   a) Change unpredictably in sign and size
   b) Remain constant or vary predictably
   c) Are always positive
   d) Cannot be reduced by calibration

11. Gross errors are best handled by:

    a) Averaging all readings
    b) Excluding obvious outliers from analysis
    c) Applying statistical weighting
    d) Increasing measurement frequency

12. Random errors can be reduced by:

    a) Calibration of the instrument
    b) Taking the mean of many repeated measurements
    c) Substituting instruments
    d) Changing measurement units

13. The mean of a dataset indicates:

    a) Dispersion of data
    b) Central tendency of values
    c) Frequency of outliers
    d) Measurement bias

14. The variance is:

    a) The square of the mean
    b) The second central moment
    c) The mean absolute deviation
    d) The reciprocal of standard deviation

15. The standard deviation (σ) quantifies:

    a) Average value
    b) Uncertainty due to random fluctuations
    c) Instrumental bias
    d) Measurement resolution

16. The normal (Gaussian) distribution assumes:

    a) Only positive deviations occur
    b) Large deviations are more frequent than small ones
    c) Positive and negative deviations occur equally often
    d) Mean $\neq$ Median

17. The 68–95–99.7 rule for a normal distribution means that approximately:

    a) 68%, 95%, and 99.7% of data lie within 1σ, 2σ, and 3σ of the mean
    b) 68% of data lie outside 3σ
    c) 95% of data equal the mean
    d) 99.7% of data are errors

18. The Student's t-distribution is primarily used when:

    a) Population variance is unknown and sample size is small
    b) Data are uniformly distributed
    c) Measurements are categorical
    d) Variance is zero

19. The chi-square distribution is applied to:

    a) Test equality of two means
    b) Evaluate variances and goodness-of-fit
    c) Measure systematic bias
    d) Calculate relative error

20. The F-distribution is used to:

    a) Compare two variances
    b) Determine standard deviation
    c) Estimate population mean
    d) Remove gross errors

21. Intrinsic errors occur:

    a) Under ideal laboratory conditions only
    b) Under normal operating conditions of an instrument
    c) Only when external interference exists
    d) Due to human reading mistakes

22. Dynamic errors arise because:

    a) Instruments respond instantaneously
    b) The measurement system has finite response time
    c) Calibration was repeated too often
    d) Environmental temperature is constant

23. Preventive measures for reducing systematic error include:

    a) Substitution and reversal methods during measurement
    b) Thermal stabilization and calibration before use
    c) Applying correction coefficients after measurement
    d) Ignoring environmental changes

24. The main goal of normalization of metrological characteristics is to:

    a) Guarantee consistent accuracy under expected conditions
    b) Reduce operator workload
    c) Eliminate random noise entirely
    d) Simplify statistical calculations

25. A series of five repeated measurements of a voltage yields the following values (V): 1.02, 1.05, 1.00, 1.03, 0.98.

   a) Determine the mean value.
   b) Compute the standard deviation (σ).
   c) If the conventional true value is 1.00 V, calculate the absolute and relative errors for the mean measurement.

4.2.4   ISO GUM and Uncertainty Budgeting in Biosensors

1. Measurement uncertainty expresses:

   a) The exact difference between measured and true value
   b) The range within which the true value is believed to lie
   c) The number of significant figures in a reading
   d) The smallest detectable signal

2. The primary international framework defining uncertainty evaluation is:

   a) ISO 15197
   b) ISO GUM (Guide to the Expression of Uncertainty in Measurement)
   c) ISO 9001
   d) IEC 61010

3. In biosensor measurements, uncertainty is crucial because it:

   a) Determines electrode geometry
   b) Quantifies confidence in the reported result
   c) Eliminates all random errors
   d) Ensures identical readings across laboratories

4. Error differs from uncertainty because:

   a) Error is a range; uncertainty is a single value
   b) Error is deviation from the true value, uncertainty is doubt about it
   c) Error can be completely eliminated
   d) Uncertainty depends only on calibration

5. The measurand in biosensor analysis must be:

   a) Implicitly defined by the device manufacturer
   b) Clearly and completely defined to ensure comparability
   c) Independent of environmental conditions
   d) Expressed in arbitrary units

6. An incomplete definition of the measurand leads to:

   a) Improved reproducibility
   b) Ambiguity and added uncertainty
   c) Lower systematic error
   d) Faster measurement speed

7. Random errors in biosensors originate mainly from:

   a) Calibration bias
   b) Electronic noise and biological variability
   c) Incorrect reference values
   d) Operator bias

8. Systematic errors are characterized by:

   a) Unpredictable magnitude and direction
   b) Consistent deviation caused by repeatable influences
   c) Random sign changes between trials
   d) Reduction through averaging only

9. In biosensors, a consistent offset due to reference-electrode aging is an example of:

   a) Random error
   b) Systematic error
   c) Gross error
   d) Type B uncertainty

10. The distinction between error and uncertainty is important because:

    a) It identifies the measurand's molecular weight
    b) It prevents misinterpretation of biosensor accuracy
    c) It removes calibration requirements
    d) It simplifies signal processing

11. Influence quantities in biosensors include:

    a) Temperature, pH, flow rate, and electrode condition
    b) Only analyte concentration
    c) Manufacturer batch number
    d) Data-logging frequency

12. Measurement uncertainty in biosensors is expressed as:

    a) Error percentage only
    b) A parameter, often a standard deviation or a multiple of it
    c) A qualitative estimate without statistics
    d) A unit-less coefficient of variation

13. The **standard uncertainty (u)** represents:

   a) The expanded uncertainty at 95% confidence
   b) The standard deviation associated with a measured value
   c) The mean of repeated results
   d) The bias of the instrument

14. The **expanded uncertainty (U)** is calculated as:

   a) $U = u/k$
   b) $U = k \times u$
   c) $U = \sqrt{k/u}$
   d) $U = k + u$

15. A coverage factor $k = 2$ corresponds approximately to a confidence level of:

   a) 68%
   b) 90%
   c) 95%
   d) 99%

16. Type A evaluation of uncertainty is based on:

   a) Statistical analysis of repeated measurements
   b) Manufacturer specifications only
   c) Expert judgment
   d) Calibration certificates

17. The standard uncertainty of the mean is calculated as:

   a) $u = s \times \sqrt{n}$
   b) $u = s/\sqrt{n}$
   c) $u = 1/(s \times n)$
   d) $u = n/s$

18. Type B evaluation uses information from:

   a) Repeatability tests only
   b) Previous data, calibration certificates, or expert judgment
   c) Random error analysis
   d) Student's t-distribution

19. For a rectangular (uniform) distribution with half-width $\pm a$, the standard uncertainty is:

   a) $a/\sqrt{2}$
   b) $a/\sqrt{3}$
   c) $a/\sqrt{6}$
   d) $a/2$

20. If an instrument specification states ±0.4 mV with 95% confidence (normal distribution), the standard uncertainty u is approximately:

    a) $0.4/2 = 0.2$ mV
    b) $0.4/1.96 \approx 0.204$ mV
    c) $0.4 \times 2 = 0.8$ mV
    d) $0.4 \times 1.96 = 0.784$ mV

21. The combined standard uncertainty $u\_c(Y)$ is obtained by:

    a) Adding all errors algebraically
    b) Using the root-sum-square of individual components
    c) Multiplying all uncertainties
    d) Taking the largest uncertainty only

22. The effective degrees of freedom (v_eff) are estimated using the:

    a) Gauss–Markov equation
    b) Welch–Satterthwaite equation
    c) Bayes theorem
    d) Fourier series expansion

23. When reporting uncertainty, significant figures should:

    a) Include as many decimals as possible
    b) Reflect measurement precision with at most two significant digits for U
    c) Be independent of U
    d) Match the instrument's display digits

24. The main elements of a biosensor traceability chain include:

    a) Reference materials, instrument calibration, environmental monitoring, and documentation
    b) Sample storage and labeling only
    c) Data encryption systems
    d) Randomized operator selection

25. A biosensor yields five repeated current readings (μA): 9.8, 10.1, 10.0, 9.9, 10.2.

    a) Compute the mean and standard deviation (s).
    b) Determine the standard uncertainty of the mean $u = s/\sqrt{n}$.
    c) If $k = 2$, find the expanded uncertainty $U = k \times u$ and express the result as $Y = y \pm U$ (95% confidence).

4.2.5   Electrochemical Biosensors

1. An electrochemical biosensor primarily converts a biological interaction into:

   a) A thermal gradient
   b) An optical emission
   c) An electrical signal
   d) A color change

2. The component responsible for selective analyte recognition in a biosensor is the:

   a) Electrode surface
   b) Transducer
   c) Biological recognition element
   d) Signal processor

3. Disposable electrochemical biosensors are preferred when:

   a) Recalibration is impossible
   b) Sterility and contamination control are critical
   c) Signal amplification is unnecessary
   d) Continuous monitoring is required

4. Which of the following best distinguishes catalytic from affinity biosensors?

   a) Catalytic sensors involve equilibrium binding; affinity sensors use enzyme reactions
   b) Catalytic sensors rely on enzymatic reactions; affinity sensors depend on binding events
   c) Both depend solely on temperature stability
   d) There is no distinction

5. According to IUPAC, biosensor performance should be characterized by:

   a) Linearity, precision, and selectivity
   b) Only the detection limit
   c) Visual response time
   d) Sample color change

6. Point-of-care electrochemical biosensors are designed primarily for:

   a) Industrial synthesis
   b) Bedside or on-site testing
   c) Environmental storage
   d) Long-term incubation

7. The biological event in a biosensor is transformed into an electrical signal by the:

   a) Amplifier
   b) Transducer
   c) Reference electrode
   d) Enzyme

8. In early biosensor history, physical instruments such as thermometers were misclassified because:

   a) They lacked biological recognition elements
   b) They were optical devices
   c) They contained electrodes
   d) They were temperature dependent

9. The first enzyme-based electrochemical biosensor was inspired by:

   a) The hydrogen electrode
   b) Clark's oxygen electrode (1956)
   c) The glass pH electrode
   d) The photodiode array

10. Electrochemical biosensors can be grouped mainly as:

   a) Optical and mechanical
   b) Biocatalytic and affinity-based
   c) Conductive and photometric
   d) Chromatic and enzymatic

11. The **working electrode** in an electrochemical biosensor:

   a) Maintains constant potential
   b) Provides the site for biochemical interaction and signal generation
   c) Balances system current
   d) Amplifies the output

12. The **reference electrode** serves to:

   a) Stabilize current flow
   b) Maintain a fixed potential for accurate measurement
   c) Generate biochemical reactions
   d) Filter electrical noise

13. **Ag/AgCl** reference electrodes may lose accuracy due to:

   a) Chloride ion depletion
   b) Protein adsorption
   c) High humidity
   d) Electrode oxidation by air

14. A **potentiostat** maintains:

    a) Constant current between working and counter electrodes
    b) Constant potential between working and reference electrodes
    c) Constant impedance across all electrodes
    d) Constant frequency response

15. A **galvanostat** differs from a potentiostat in that it:

    a) Controls potential rather than current
    b) Controls current rather than potential
    c) Measures impedance spectra
    d) Operates without electrodes

16. The Nernst equation is essential because it relates:

    a) Temperature and pressure
    b) Electrode potential to reactant concentration
    c) Magnetic field to current
    d) Enzyme concentration to viscosity

17. The overall current response in an electrochemical biosensor depends on:

    a) Analyte diffusion, applied potential, and reaction kinetics
    b) Light absorption and temperature alone
    c) Mechanical stress in electrodes
    d) Only the electrode area

18. The potential difference measured by potentiometric biosensors arises from:

    a) Ion-selective changes at the electrode interface
    b) Optical emission
    c) Gas bubble formation
    d) Temperature fluctuations

19. A glucose biosensor produces 8.5 µA at 2.0 mM and 17 µA at 4.0 mM glucose.

    a) Determine the slope (sensitivity) in $\mu A\ mM^{-1}$.
    b) Predict the current at 6.0 mM assuming linearity.
    c) If baseline noise is ±0.5 µA, estimate the limit of detection (LOD $\approx 3 \times$ noise/slope).

20. A urea biosensor shows a 58 mV potential change per decade of concentration at 25 °C.

    a) What is the expected slope at 37 °C (298 K → 310 K)?
    b) Calculate the theoretical slope from the Nernst relation ($RT/nF \times 2.303$) for $n = 1$ and compare.

4.2.6   Optical Biosensors

1. Optical biosensors detect biological interactions primarily through changes in:

   a) Voltage and current
   b) Light intensity or wavelength
   c) Mechanical vibration
   d) Thermal gradients

2. The biorecognition element in an optical biosensor provides:

   a) Signal amplification
   b) Specific analyte binding
   c) Data interpretation
   d) Temperature control

3. The transducer in an optical biosensor converts:

   a) Light into mechanical motion
   b) Biological events into optical signals
   c) Electrical signals into light
   d) Temperature into color

4. Typical optical signals monitored in biosensors include:

   a) Voltage, current, resistance
   b) Intensity, wavelength, polarization, refractive index
   c) pH and temperature
   d) Acoustic wave frequency

5. The first enzyme-based biosensor was developed by:

   a) Michaelis and Menten
   b) Leland C. Clark Jr. and Champ Lyons
   c) Fred Sanger
   d) Linus Pauling

6. Surface plasmon resonance (SPR) detects:

   a) Temperature fluctuations
   b) Changes in refractive index near a metal surface
   c) Chemical luminescence
   d) Gas pressure

7. The 1990s were a turning point for optical biosensors due to the introduction of:

   a) DNA sequencing
   b) Surface plasmon resonance and fluorescent proteins
   c) Nanoparticles
   d) Quantum computing

8. Immobilization of biological molecules in optical biosensors is critical because it:

   a) Reduces signal-to-noise ratio
   b) Maintains biological activity and stability
   c) Increases color intensity
   d) Prevents fluorescence

9. Which immobilization technique involves covalent bonding to a surface?

   a) Adsorption
   b) Entrapment
   c) Cross-linking
   d) Covalent attachment

10. Cell-based optical biosensors are particularly useful in:

    a) Measuring light polarization
    b) Toxicity and pharmacological testing
    c) DNA sequencing
    d) Colorimetric assays

11. Fluorescence biosensors operate on the principle that:

    a) Absorbed light produces electrical current
    b) Excited fluorophores emit light at longer wavelengths
    c) Light intensity remains constant
    d) Heat alters color

12. Interferometric biosensors detect analyte binding by measuring:

    a) Current flow
    b) Optical path differences between two beams
    c) Enzyme reaction rates
    d) Sound wave amplitude

13. Colorimetric biosensors depend on:

    a) Fluorescent protein expression
    b) Visible color changes upon analyte binding
    c) Raman signal intensity
    d) Refractive index variations

14. The dynamic range of an optical biosensor refers to:

    a) The voltage range of detection
    b) The minimum and maximum detectable analyte concentrations
    c) The lifetime of the biosensor
    d) The optical wavelength span

15. Laser diodes are used when:

   a) Monochromatic and coherent light is required
   b) A diffuse light source is sufficient
   c) Only visual detection is needed
   d) Wide-spectrum emission is desired

16. Photodiodes convert:

   a) Electrical energy into photons
   b) Light into electrical current
   c) Sound into voltage
   d) Heat into luminescence

17. CCD and CMOS detectors are primarily used for:

   a) Temperature stabilization
   b) Imaging and high-throughput fluorescence analysis
   c) Controlling light polarization
   d) Mechanical calibration

18. Amplifiers and filters in biosensor circuits serve to:

   a) Enhance weak optical signals and remove noise
   b) Change light color
   c) Convert current to pH
   d) Store data only

19. Signal preprocessing in optical biosensors often involves:

   a) Image distortion and stretching
   b) Filtering, baseline correction, and normalization
   c) Random noise addition
   d) Manual data entry

20. The function of a GUI (Graphical User Interface) is to:

   a) Regulate optical fiber temperature
   b) Provide user-friendly visualization and control
   c) Generate light pulses
   d) Analyze Raman spectra automatically

4.2.7   Impedance Biosensors

1. Electrochemical impedance spectroscopy (EIS) investigates system behavior by:

   a) Applying a steady potential and measuring current decay
   b) Applying an AC signal and analyzing voltage–current phase response

   c) Recording temperature variation over time

   d) Measuring charge accumulation only

2. Impedance differs from resistance because it:

   a) Has both magnitude and phase components

   b) Depends only on DC voltage

   c) Is purely real

   d) Cannot be frequency-dependent

3. Transforming time-domain data into frequency-domain spectra enables:

   a) Elimination of capacitive effects

   b) Separation of simultaneous electrochemical processes

   c) Noise-free measurements

   d) Current amplification

4. Compared with cyclic voltammetry, EIS provides:

   a) Less information on kinetics

   b) Frequency-resolved insight into charge transfer and diffusion

   c) Instantaneous potential scans

   d) Only steady-state values

5. The concept of impedance as a diffusion-related function was introduced by:

   a) Oliver Heaviside

   b) Erich Warburg

   c) Walther Nernst

   d) Michael Faraday

6. The invention that enabled precise electrode-potential control was the:

   a) Galvanometer

   b) Potentiostat

   c) Thermocouple

   d) Wheatstone bridge

7. The Warburg impedance models:

   a) Charge transfer

   b) Diffusion-controlled processes

   c) Double-layer charging

   d) Electrode corrosion

8. The standard EIS electrode configuration includes:

   a) Two identical reference electrodes

   b) Working, reference, and counter electrodes

   c) Two counter electrodes

   d) Photodiode and anode

9. Surface modification with gold nanoparticles or graphene primarily improves:

   a) Color visibility
   b) Electroactive area and conductivity
   c) pH buffering
   d) Thermal insulation

10. A Randles circuit typically contains:

    a) Two capacitors in parallel
    b) Rs, Rct, Cdl, and Zw elements
    c) Only Rct and Rs
    d) Inductive and magnetic components only

11. A Nyquist plot of an ideal Randles cell shows:

    a) A straight line through the origin
    b) A semicircle followed by a 45° tail
    c) Random scatter
    d) A horizontal plateau

12. Conductometric biosensors measure:

    a) Voltage changes
    b) Solution conductivity variations
    c) Optical intensity
    d) Temperature fluctuations

13. Potentiometric biosensors rely on detecting:

    a) Electrical potential differences due to ion activity
    b) Current flow
    c) Mechanical stress
    d) Absorbance

14. Amperometric biosensors quantify analyte concentration by:

    a) Measuring current from redox reactions
    b) Recording light emission
    c) Calculating impedance angles
    d) Measuring resistance only

15. Impedimetric biosensors differ because they:

    a) Require fluorescent labels
    b) Measure changes in complex impedance caused by molecular binding
    c) Operate without electrodes
    d) Detect temperature

16. Portable EIS devices are valuable for:

    a) Long-term laboratory experiments only
    b) Point-of-care and field diagnostics
    c) Nuclear research
    d) Optical analysis alone

17. Wearable EIS biosensors commonly monitor:

    a) Atmospheric pressure
    b) Sweat biomarkers like glucose or lactate
    c) Sound waves
    d) Electrical resistance in metals

18. Implantable EIS devices must prioritize:

    a) High temperature operation
    b) Biocompatibility and wireless communication
    c) Large battery packs
    d) Optical excitation

19. In cancer diagnostics, EIS biosensors can detect:

    a) HER2, PSA, CEA tumor biomarkers
    b) Only red blood cells
    c) ATP synthesis rate
    d) MRI signals

20. Cardiovascular EIS biosensors measure biomarkers such as:

    a) Troponin and CRP
    b) Hemoglobin and bilirubin
    c) Lactate dehydrogenase only
    d) Urea and creatinine

4.2.8   Acoustic and Piezoelectric Biosensors

1. Acoustic and piezoelectric biosensors operate based on:

    a) The photoelectric effect
    b) The piezoelectric effect
    c) The thermoelectric effect
    d) The electrochemical redox effect

2. The piezoelectric effect involves:

   a) Emission of photons when a crystal is heated
   b) Generation of electric charge by mechanical stress
   c) Magnetic alignment of dipoles
   d) Absorption of sound energy

3. QCM and SAW sensors detect:

   a) Optical reflection changes
   b) Variations in mass or viscoelastic properties on the surface
   c) Changes in electrode current
   d) Temperature gradients in a crystal

4. Acoustic biosensors are often preferred because they:

   a) Require fluorescent labeling
   b) Operate label-free and in real time
   c) Depend on external catalysts
   d) Only function in gaseous media

5. Integration of microfluidic systems with QCM and SAW sensors allows:

   a) Reduced control over sample handling
   b) Automated, multiplexed, and low-volume analyses
   c) Elimination of signal processing
   d) Manual calibration only

6. The oxygen electrode, regarded as the first biosensor, was invented by:

   a) Walther Nernst
   b) Leland C. Clark Jr.
   c) Erich Warburg
   d) Hans Berger

7. The QCM measures:

   a) Changes in current
   b) Changes in resonant frequency due to mass variations
   c) Voltage shifts due to pH
   d) Color intensity of samples

8. The fundamental QCM frequency $f_0 = \dfrac{n}{2t_q}\sqrt{\dfrac{\mu_q}{\rho_q}}$ depends on:

   a) Crystal radius
   b) Shear modulus, density, and thickness
   c) Refractive index
   d) Surface tension

9. According to the Sauerbrey relation, an increase in surface mass causes:

   a) Frequency increase
   b) Frequency decrease

c) Voltage increase
d) Resistance increase

10. The Sauerbrey constant C depends on:

   a) Electrode material
   b) Crystal parameters and geometry
   c) Solution viscosity
   d) Measurement temperature only

11. The AT-cut quartz crystal is oriented at approximately:

   a) $10°$ to the z-axis
   b) $35°25'$ to the z-axis
   c) $45°$ to the z-axis
   d) $90°$ to the z-axis

12. The QCM typically oscillates in the:

   a) Longitudinal compression mode
   b) Thickness shear mode
   c) Flexural bending mode
   d) Torsional mode

13. Common electrode materials for QCM fabrication include:

   a) Silver and nickel
   b) Gold and platinum
   c) Chromium and iron
   d) Copper and aluminum

14. SAW sensors detect changes through:

   a) Propagation of electromagnetic radiation
   b) Acoustic wave modulation along a piezoelectric surface
   c) Diffusion of ions in an electrolyte
   d) Optical reflectance

15. The key components of a SAW device include:

   a) Electrodes, thermistors, and magnets
   b) Piezoelectric substrate and interdigital transducers (IDTs)
   c) Glass plates and optical fibers
   d) Microfluidic valves only

16. In delay-line SAW sensors, the acoustic wave:

   a) Is confined between reflective gratings
   b) Propagates freely between input and output IDTs
   c) Is absorbed by a liquid layer
   d) Converts into heat

17. In resonator-type SAW sensors, acoustic energy is:

   a) Dissipated immediately
   b) Confined between two reflective gratings
   c) Amplified by a photodiode
   d) Converted to fluorescence

18. In QCM and SAW biosensors, the transducer converts:

   a) Chemical energy to heat
   b) Biological interactions into mechanical or electrical signals
   c) Sound to light
   d) Voltage to optical intensity

19. In QCM biosensors, a frequency decrease indicates:

   a) Surface erosion
   b) Mass accumulation due to analyte binding
   c) Increased voltage
   d) Temperature rise

20. SAW biosensors are particularly sensitive because:

   a) Acoustic waves penetrate deeply into the substrate
   b) Acoustic waves are confined near the surface
   c) They rely on magnetic resonance
   d) They use chemical amplification

4.2.9   Electrical and Field-Effect Biosensors

1. A biosensor typically contains which four core components?

   a) Analyte, bioreceptor, transducer, processor
   b) Sample, filter, amplifier, display
   c) Catalyst, battery, sensor chip, heater
   d) Buffer, optical lens, electrode, screen

2. Modern biosensors detect analytes by converting biological recognition into:

   a) Optical patterns
   b) Electrical or mechanical signals
   c) Thermal gradients
   d) Acoustic waves only

3. Electrical biosensors are widely used in:

   a) Clinical diagnostics and environmental testing
   b) Astronomical observations

   c) Marine navigation
   d) Food color enhancement

4. The measurable signal in an electrical biosensor most often arises from changes in:

   a) Light scattering
   b) Current, voltage, or impedance
   c) Magnetic induction
   d) Temperature gradient

5. The three electrodes in a FET are:

   a) Anode, cathode, and reference
   b) Source, drain, and gate
   c) Emitter, collector, and base
   d) Cathode, ground, and shield

6. The semiconducting channel conducts current between:

   a) Source and drain
   b) Gate and substrate
   c) Electrolyte and reference
   d) Cathode and anode

7. The dielectric layer in BioFETs is commonly made of:

   a) SiO_2, Al_2O_3, or HfO_2
   b) Polyethylene or nylon
   c) Gold or silver
   d) Carbon paste

8. The function of the buffer in a BioFET system is to:

   a) Supply power to the device
   b) Maintain physiological conditions and enable ion exchange
   c) Block light interference
   d) Increase viscosity

9. The oxide capacitance per unit area (C_{ox}) affects:

   a) Electrode adhesion
   b) Threshold voltage shift (ΔV_T)
   c) Signal visualization
   d) Noise filtering

10. The Ag/AgCl electrode in a liquid-gate FET acts as the:

   a) Source electrode
   b) Reference gate electrode
   c) Current sink
   d) Substrate holder

11. Amperometric biosensors measure:

   a) Current from redox reactions
   b) Potential under zero current
   c) Capacitance
   d) Acoustic frequency

12. Potentiometric biosensors are commonly used for:

   a) Pressure measurement
   b) pH and ion detection
   c) Gas flow control
   d) Color change analysis

13. Conductometric biosensors operate by detecting changes in:

   a) Solution conductivity
   b) Magnetic flux
   c) Optical absorbance
   d) Pressure

14. Capacitive biosensors are particularly suited for:

   a) Monitoring protein binding events
   b) Counting cells in suspension
   c) Thermal profiling
   d) Magnetic particle alignment

15. Impedimetric biosensors measure:

   a) Voltage gain
   b) Total impedance (resistance + reactance)
   c) Power loss
   d) pH fluctuations

16. The ISFET detects changes in:

   a) Light intensity
   b) Ion concentration, especially H^+ (pH)
   c) Temperature
   d) Flow rate

17. The Enzyme FET (EnFET) monitors:

   a) Gas composition
   b) Ionic changes caused by enzymatic reactions
   c) Mechanical stress
   d) Radiation intensity

18. The ImmunoFET relies on:

   a) Antibody-antigen binding altering surface charge

   b) Optical absorption
   c) Magnetic dipole alignment
   d) Temperature-induced current flow

19. The DNA-FET detects:

   a) Hydrogen bond lengths by spectroscopy
   b) Nucleic acid hybridization via charge density change
   c) Optical fluorescence
   d) Thermal conductivity

20. Cell-based BioFETs measure:

   a) Cellular membrane potential and metabolic activity
   b) Cell mass only
   c) Optical refractive index
   d) Protein fluorescence

4.2.10   *Immunosensors*

1. Immunosensors detect biomolecules through:

   a) Electrochemical redox reactions only
   b) Specific antibody–antigen interactions
   c) Mechanical compression
   d) Temperature-dependent diffusion

2. The measurable signal in an immunosensor originates from:

   a) Non-specific protein adsorption
   b) Formation of an immunocomplex between antibody and antigen
   c) Electrolysis of the analyte
   d) Sample evaporation

3. Electrochemical immunosensors are widely used because they:

   a) Require expensive optical setups
   b) Are sensitive, portable, and easily miniaturized
   c) Operate only at high voltages
   d) Depend solely on light intensity

4. Modern immunosensors are valuable for detecting:

   a) Only glucose and urea
   b) Cancer biomarkers, infectious agents, and therapeutic drugs
   c) pH and conductivity
   d) Only physical parameters

5. A major advantage of immunosensors over traditional assays is their:

   a) Requirement for large reagent volumes
   b) Real-time and label-free detection capability
   c) Inability to quantify analytes
   d) Dependence on complex sample preparation

6. The key components of an immunosensor include:

   a) Battery, resistor, amplifier
   b) Biorecognition element, transducer, signal processor
   c) Enzyme, light source, microfilter
   d) Reagent reservoir, heater, cooler

7. The biorecognition element ensures:

   a) Selectivity toward the target analyte
   b) Mechanical stability
   c) Temperature control
   d) Data storage

8. The transducer converts:

   a) Chemical reactions into thermal noise
   b) Biological recognition into measurable physical signals
   c) Electrical signals into photons
   d) Mechanical vibration into enzyme activity

9. Among transducer types, electrochemical ones are favored because of:

   a) High sensitivity and low cost
   b) Light absorption properties
   c) Large sample volume requirement
   d) Incompatibility with miniaturization

10. Piezoelectric transducers detect changes in:

    a) Voltage drop
    b) Mass or elasticity on the sensor surface
    c) Temperature gradient
    d) Light wavelength

11. Optical transducers detect variations in:

    a) Refractive index, fluorescence, or absorbance
    b) Ion concentration only
    c) Mechanical resonance
    d) Voltage bias

12. Antibodies are preferred in immunosensors because:

    a) They are inexpensive but non-selective
    b) They offer high specificity for target antigens

   c) They are chemically inert and conductive
   d) They eliminate calibration needs

13. Aptamers differ from antibodies by being:

   a) Synthetic oligonucleotides with tunable stability
   b) Large polysaccharides
   c) Magnetic nanoparticles
   d) Protein-based enzymes

14. Molecularly imprinted polymers (MIPs) provide:

   a) Natural receptor binding only
   b) Synthetic recognition sites mimicking biological targets
   c) Enzymatic catalysis
   d) Poor reproducibility

15. Peptides are used in immunosensors because they:

   a) Provide lower selectivity than antibodies
   b) Can mimic antibody binding sites and are easy to synthesize
   c) Are unstable in all buffers
   d) Require labeling for every use

16. Key performance metrics for immunosensors include:

   a) Sensitivity, specificity, stability, and response time
   b) Voltage bias and optical power
   c) Temperature drift and pressure drop
   d) Color intensity only

17. Amperometric immunosensors measure:

   a) Potential difference
   b) Current produced by redox reactions
   c) Temperature changes
   d) Refractive index

18. Potentiometric immunosensors are characterized by:

   a) Measuring electrode potential changes
   b) Measuring mechanical deformation
   c) Measuring light emission
   d) Measuring thermal conductivity

19. Impedimetric immunosensors detect:

   a) Impedance changes at the electrode interface
   b) Color shifts in the medium
   c) Acoustic waves
   d) Enzyme fluorescence

20. Quartz Crystal Microbalance (QCM) immunosensors measure:

    a) Temperature rise
    b) Frequency shifts proportional to bound mass
    c) Potential difference
    d) Light polarization

21. Thermometric immunosensors detect:

    a) Refractive index
    b) Temperature changes from exothermic or endothermic reactions
    c) Pressure
    d) Voltage gain

22. Immunosensors are crucial for detecting biomarkers in:

    a) Soil samples only
    b) Cancer, infectious diseases, and autoimmune disorders
    c) Optical fiber networks
    d) Electrical grids

23. Common tumor markers analyzed using immunosensors include:

    a) PSA, CEA, AFP
    b) Hemoglobin and bilirubin
    c) Creatinine and urea
    d) Dopamine and serotonin

24. Autoimmune disorders diagnosed using immunosensors may involve detection of:

    a) Anti-nuclear antibodies (ANA) and rheumatoid factor (RF)
    b) Blood glucose
    c) Iron levels
    d) Magnesium ions

25. In therapeutic drug monitoring, immunosensors are used to:

    a) Adjust drug dosage by measuring concentration in biological fluids
    b) Measure tissue temperature
    c) Estimate drug solubility only
    d) Detect optical density

4.2.11   Biomedical Applications of Biosensors

1. Biomedical biosensors measure biological changes by coupling:

    a) A mechanical transducer with a heat sensor
    b) A biological recognition element with a physical transducer

   c) A magnetic probe with a photodiode

   d) A pressure gauge with a microfilter

2. The biological recognition element in a biosensor may include:

   a) Enzyme, antibody, nucleic acid, or living cell

   b) Battery, resistor, or switch

   c) Optical fiber, LED, or screen

   d) Metallic alloy only

3. Biosensors are primarily used in medicine for:

   a) Color correction and image processing

   b) Disease diagnosis and patient monitoring

   c) Magnetic resonance imaging

   d) Ultrasound calibration

4. One major benefit of biosensors over traditional assays is:

   a) Higher reagent consumption

   b) Slower analysis time

   c) Faster, more portable detection

   d) Requirement for large sample volumes

5. Continuous glucose monitoring (CGM) devices are examples of:

   a) Colorimetric biosensors

   b) Implantable or wearable electrochemical biosensors

   c) Optical-only detectors

   d) Genetic sequencing platforms

6. Optical biosensors such as SPR are useful for detecting:

   a) Mechanical strain

   b) Cancer biomarkers like PSA or HER2

   c) Bacterial motility

   d) Light intensity fluctuations only

7. The detection principle of Surface Plasmon Resonance (SPR) involves:

   a) Current flow in an enzyme electrode

   b) Refractive-index changes upon biomolecular binding

   c) Magnetic induction

   d) Optical absorption by metal salts

8. HER2 is an important biomarker in:

   a) Prostate cancer

   b) Breast cancer

   c) Ovarian cancer

   d) Leukemia

9. Compared with PCR, nucleic-acid biosensors offer:

   a) Longer analysis times
   b) Rapid, field-deployable testing
   c) Dependence on thermocyclers
   d) Low specificity

10. A genosensor operates by detecting:

   a) Nucleotide sequence hybridization
   b) Thermal conductivity
   c) Color contrast
   d) Electrostatic discharge

11. The detection limit of an advanced optical biosensor for HER2 may reach:

   a) $1\ \mu g/mL$
   b) $0.01\ ng/mL$
   c) $1\ mg/mL$
   d) $1\ \mu M$

12. Implantable biosensors can directly:

   a) Measure tissue biomarkers and control drug delivery
   b) Record sound waves
   c) Track blood pressure optically
   d) Measure mechanical force

13. The artificial-pancreas system integrates:

   a) Optical detection of lactate
   b) Biosensor with an insulin pump for closed-loop control
   c) DNA sequencing chip
   d) Heart-rate monitor

14. Optical biosensors in smartwatches use which principle?

   a) Photoplethysmography (PPG)
   b) Piezoelectric resonance
   c) Electrochemical oxidation
   d) Capacitance change

15. Wireless data transmission in wearable sensors enables:

   a) Direct physician access for real-time monitoring
   b) Manual data logging only
   c) Random data loss prevention
   d) Faster chemical reactions

16. Biosensors integrated with EEG or ECG systems help detect:

   a) Arrhythmias, seizures, and sleep disorders

   b) Optical fluorescence
   c) Antigen–antibody reactions
   d) Blood pH

17. Preventive biosensors detecting CRP can help identify:

   a) Cancer metastasis
   b) Inflammatory or infectious diseases early
   c) Blood viscosity changes
   d) Genetic mutations

18. Artificial-intelligence integration in biosensors enables:

   a) Predictive analytics and noise reduction
   b) Data deletion
   c) Manual reading interpretation
   d) Optical excitation control

19. IoT-connected biosensors allow:

   a) Real-time communication with healthcare networks
   b) Data storage only on the device
   c) Offline analysis only
   d) Magnetic power supply

20. Predictive algorithms in AI-based biosensors can:

   a) Forecast glucose fluctuations or cardiac stress
   b) Alter enzyme kinetics
   c) Change pH of samples
   d) Eliminate calibration procedures

9783032157560